DEDICATIONS

Sue Hinchliff – To my daughter Katy, a nurse of whom I am very proud!
Sally Thomson – For Bill and Gilly
Dave Barton – To Jan and the boys
Sue Howard – To James, Alex and Ben

Commissioning Editor: Steven Black, Mairi McCubbin
Development Editor: Carole McMurray
Project Manager: Anne Dickie and Srikumar Narayanan
Designer: George Ajayi
Illustration Manager: Merlyn Harvey
Illustrator: David Banks

The Practitioner as Teacher

Fourth Edition

Edited by

Sue Hinchliff BA MSc RN RNT
Visiting Professor of Nursing and Nurse Education, London South Bank University,
Consultant to Royal College of Nursing Accreditation Unit,
Consultant to Nursing and Midwifery Council in Advanced Nursing Practice,
Adviser to Tropical Health and Education Trust

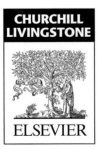

CHURCHILL
LIVINGSTONE

ELSEVIER

EDINBURGH LONDON NEW YORK OXFORD PHILADELPHIA ST LOUIS SYDNEY TORONTO 2009

CHURCHILL
LIVINGSTONE
ELSEVIER

First published 1991
Second edition 1999
Third edition 2004
Fourth edition 2009
  Reprinted 2010

ISBN: 978 0 7020 2999 8

British Library Cataloguing in Publication Data
A catalogue record for this book is available from the British Library

Library of Congress Cataloging in Publication Data
A catalog record for this book is available from the Library of Congress

Notice
Knowledge and best practice in this field are constantly changing. As new research and experience broaden our knowledge, changes in practice, treatment and drug therapy may become necessary or appropriate. Readers are advised to check the most current information provided (i) on procedures featured or (ii) by the manufacturer of each product to be administered, to verify the recommended dose or formula, the method and duration of administration, and contraindications. It is the responsibility of the practitioner, relying on their own experience and knowledge of the patient, to make diagnoses, to determine dosages and the best treatment for each individual patient, and to take all appropriate safety precautions. To the fullest extent of the law, neither the Publisher nor the Authors assume any liability for any injury and/or damage to persons or property arising out of or related to any use of the material contained in this book.

The Publisher

The
Publisher's
policy is to use
**paper manufactured
from sustainable forests**

Printed in China

Contents

Contents

List of contributors

TD Barton PhD MPhil BEd DipN RGN RNT
Academic Lead for the Department of Nursing, School of Health Science, Faculty of Health and Human Sciences, Swansea University/Prifysgol Abertawe Singleton Park, Swansea, UK

Sue Howard MA RGN DN RHV DNT Cert Ed
Healthcare Adviser, Oldham, UK

Sally Thomson RGN RMN BEd Hons MA ED
Health and Education Freelance Consultant, Kent, UK

Preface

It says a lot about the changes that have taken place in nursing and nurse education that this fourth edition of *The Practitioner as Teacher*, like the third edition, has required not just tweaks to update the text but a whole new approach.

This fourth edition is aimed at all healthcare practitioners – nurses, allied health practitioners and those who assist them – who teach in care settings. These might include hospitals, nursing homes, patients' own homes, nurse-led clinics and walk-in centres. Those who are being taught include patients, carers, other healthcare staff, peers or mentees.

The book is not pitched at a particular academic level. Rather it is designed to help anyone who has not been formally prepared as a teacher to teach others in a care setting. Nor have we set out to write an academic treatise – there are plenty of those. This is a practical, accessible 'how-to' book that sets out to give the reader some real help with teaching. We have a restricted number of references and those we have used should be readily available.

The book contains a number of activities. Readers are urged to take these seriously and to complete them. If this is done they should form a credible addition to any professional portfolio, providing evidence for:

- The Knowledge and Skills Framework (KSF) post-outline
- KSF competencies in personal and people development
- Re-registration with the Nursing and Midwifery Council
- Accreditation of Prior Experiential Learning (APEL) to gain entry on to mentoring or teaching courses
- Course work on mentoring/teaching programmes
- Appraisal and development review processes.

In a nutshell the book will help the reader to understand:

- How people learn
- How to teach
- How to use competencies
- How to support learners
- How to assess teaching and learning.

We have all enjoyed putting this text together and we hope that you will enjoy not just reading it, but *using* it! Teaching should never be dreary. It is a privilege to help someone learn; it is also gratifying, fascinating and fun.

St Albans

Sue Hinchliff

1

How we learn and how we can help others to learn

Sue Howard

Continuing professional development
- ◆ Learning environments
  Creating learning organisations and learning cultures
  Creating a learning environment for your students
- ◆ Evaluating learning
- ◆ Conclusion

INTRODUCTION

The first chapter of this book begins with two givens. The givens are that you are reading this book because you want to teach others and also that you want to know how you can better pass on your knowledge and skills to others by making your teaching more effective.

Implicit in this is the need to explore what is meant by learning and teaching in practice and also the need to understand some of the strategies that you can adopt to ensure that what you teach (and what other people learn) is also more effective.

LEARNING OBJECTIVES

After reading this chapter you should be able to:

- ◆ Understand the interdependent nature of learning and teaching

- ◆ Identify the learning theories that underpin the teaching process and apply them in practice

- ◆ Describe the different domains of learning

- ◆ Recognise the importance of individual differences in the learning process

- ◆ Identify and discuss the factors that will affect learning.

THE LEARNING–TEACHING RELATIONSHIP

If you were to ask 100 people for a definition of learning it is likely that you would get 99 different answers! This is because learning can be viewed as an activity that is quite straightforward, e.g. you have been shown how to wash your hands correctly in order to control the spread of infection, to the extremely complex, e.g., you have had an explanation of the principles of cross-infection and its effect on the patients in your care.

For the purpose of this book a very straightforward definition of learning has been used and is based on the need, in healthcare, continually to improve the standards of care given to our patients and clients. So learning is the gaining of knowledge or skills, or developing a particular behaviour, through study, instruction or experience.

So if learning is about gaining knowledge and skills, what then is teaching? Again, in this particular book we have chosen a definition that is applicable to healthcare practice. Teaching is about how we help others to gain knowledge and skills and, equally importantly, how we know that they have learned them. Central to this is the learned ability to undertake certain procedures or tasks, apparently effortlessly.

It is important to note, however, that dealing solely in definitions is sometimes problematic, as they may imply that teaching and learning are inseparable, whereas in reality it is possible for learning to take place without any noticeable teaching having occurred. This type of learning is discussed again in Chapter 2.

For this chapter, it is sufficient for us to accept that if a student is to learn, teaching in some guise is likely to have taken place – and if a teacher is to teach, there must be a student to learn. As a result, throughout this and the subsequent chapter the words 'learning' and 'teaching' will often be used interchangeably.

Another aspect of learning which is important for us to recognise is that learning can often occur over time and as a result, what we learn, in practice, becomes 'second nature'.

ACTIVITY 1.1

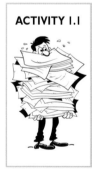

Take a few moments to think of the tasks and procedures you are able to do at work which have become 'second nature'. Now, think of everything you did on your last shift at work when you felt you were on 'automatic pilot'.

You will undoubtedly have identified numerous things that you do without being consciously aware of your actions – for example, admitting a patient to the ward or preparing someone for theatre. How we learn to undertake tasks, carry out procedures and deal with particular situations in this way is explained, in part, by different models and theories of learning and the identification of these will form the next section of the chapter.

The adult learner

New ways of learning, e.g. open, distance (sometimes now called flexible and distributed learning) and online or e-learning, have necessitated changes in the way subjects are taught. For example, traditionally, both pre-registration nursing courses and courses in continuing professional development (CPD) have been clearly structured in terms of both content and teaching strategies.

Changes in thinking about learning styles brought about, in part, by these new ways of learning have led to different approaches being used. Many of the new approaches also reflect changes which have taken place within education generally, with its increased emphasis on students under-taking projects and self-directed work. This, in turn, has led to their having different expectations about how they should be taught.

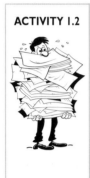

ACTIVITY 1.2

Think about a course or programme of study you have recently undertaken. Did you feel that the teaching style treated you as a child? What happened to make you feel this way? For example, the teaching style might not have been adult-centred. It could have been formal, with lots of 'chalk and talk', where the teacher decided what was to be learned. Sessions were kept strictly to time, with little or no discussion and no acknowledgement of individual learning styles within the group.

By contrast, an adult-centred session would be flexible. Recognising the needs of the individual, it would take account of different learning styles and put the student more in control of his or her learning. There would be a large element of discussion, with a degree of negotiation and an element of choice.

One of the biggest difficulties when other people are in control of our learning is that we cannot then own it. As a result, we see other people as being responsible for it. Own up! How many of you have used or heard the words 'they didn't tell me'?

Ownership of learning is fundamental to the principles of lifelong learning and it is important that, as a practitioner, you are aware of your role in ena-bling and supporting students to take responsibility for their own learning.

Andragogy and pedagogy

> The successful teacher is no longer on a height, pumping knowledge at high pressure into passive receptacles ... he is a senior student anxious to help his juniors (Sir William Osler, 1849–1919).

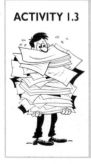

ACTIVITY 1.3

Apart from the fact that the above quotation is less gender-friendly than we would expect today, it is difficult to imagine that this was written so long ago. Reflect on what this statement means to you. How far do you agree with it? Three key issues emerge from this statement. First, effective teaching requires more than just telling someone else what you think that person ought to know. Second, the implication is that teaching is helping someone else to learn and third, teaching and learning are certainly not new phenomena.

We can look to the internet for the most straightforward definitions of andragogy and pedagogy.

Andragogy is an educational approach based on *learner*-centredness with the student's needs and wants being central to the process of teaching.

Students are responsible for, and involved in, their learning to a much greater degree than in traditional education. This can be contrasted with *pedagogy*, which is an educational approach focusing on *teacher*-centredness. The teacher is seen as an authority figure and students are not usually involved in any of the actions, or indeed decisions, regarding their learning.

(Additional very straightforward and useful definitions of teaching and learning terms can be found by accessing: www.nald.ca/adultlearningcourse/ glossary.htm.)

There are some fundamental differences in these two approaches that will ultimately affect how students learn.

Andragogy implies that:

- Learning occurs as a result of the student's own effort
- The teacher and students treat each other as equals in the teaching and learning process
- The teaching methods selected are student (or learner)-centred
- The students accept responsibility for their own learning.

Pedagogy implies that:

- Learning occurs as a result of the input of others
- The student–teacher partnership is unequal – students look up to the teacher
- Teaching methods are teacher-led
- The teacher accepts responsibility for the student's learning.

This idea is further developed by Quinn and Hughes (2007), who state that teaching can be divided into two broad categories: traditional and progressive. Traditional teaching is characterised by its teacher-centredness, with the student assuming a passive role. The progressive approach is much more student-oriented, with the student playing an active role.

ACTIVITY 1.4

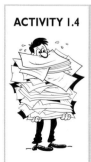

From the above, it is clear that an andragogical approach to teaching is different because it involves students being treated as adults. Think of your own experiences as a student. What led you to believe you were being treated as an adult, as opposed to the teacher having responsibility for your learning? You will probably have identified some of the following:

- There was mutual respect between you and the teacher
- Your teacher was approachable
- He or she showed a willingness to discuss rather than dictate
- The teacher accepted you as a person
- The teacher accepted your personal values.

Superficial versus deep learning

After reading this section you should be able to understand your own approach to learning and those of your students more clearly. It is a useful framework to remind you to encourage your students to become deep, as opposed to superficial learners.

Superficial learning is exactly what it implies – it is scraping the surface of the material being studied, without carrying out any deep processing of the material itself. Understanding of superficial and deep learning approaches is a very useful tool in nursing education, particularly when we consider the complex environment in which a registered nurse is required to work, as an autonomous practitioner, able to plan, implement and evaluate care using a problem-solving approach.

Deep learning requires the critical analysis of new ideas, linking them to what is already known, which in turn leads to understanding and long-term retention of concepts so that they can be used for problem-solving in unfamiliar contexts. In comparison, superficial learning involves retaining information in memory as isolated and unlinked facts. In itself it may prove to be a very useful method for undertaking examinations but it does not promote understanding or long-term retention of knowledge and information. This type of learning underpins the arguments against the use of having purely written examinations as a means of assessment, as it largely tests what an individual can remember as opposed to what the person understands.

Students who adopt a superficial approach tend to:

- Concentrate on assessment requirements (it is easy for an experienced teacher to spot this)
- Accept information and ideas passively
- Memorise facts and procedures as a matter of routine
- Ignore any patterns or guiding principles
- Fail to reflect on any underlying strategy or purpose.

Students who adopt a deep approach to learning try to turn other people's ideas into their own personalised structure of knowledge. Such students tend to:

- Try to make sense of content and issues themselves
- Be critical of the content
- Apply what is being learned to their previous knowledge and experience
- Use organising principles to integrate their ideas
- Find evidence to underpin conclusions
- Explore the logic of arguments.

Students who adopt a strategic approach to learning in this way set out with a plan of action to obtain the highest grades possible. Generally, they:

- Maintain a balanced approach to study
- Locate the right materials with which to do the work
- Are fully aware of what is required in terms of assessment criteria
- Are alert to the different roles in the student–teacher relationship.

If students are to reach their potential throughout their lifelong learning, then it is crucial to the process that they become deep learners.

The issues so far discussed, however, do not provide the whole picture as to how we learn as individuals, or indeed how it can have an influence on your teaching. Models and theories of learning provide further insight.

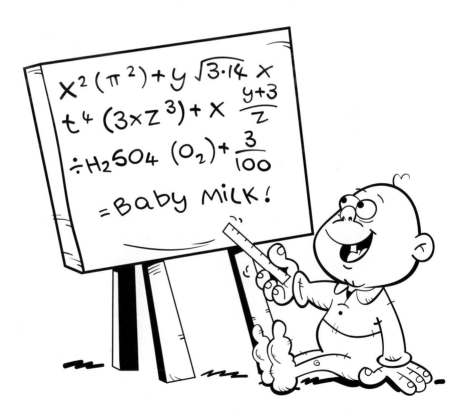

MODELS AND THEORIES OF LEARNING

If we reflect on our own learning as part of our formal education there are undoubtedly many different factors that come to mind. For example, why did some of us find it very easy to learn new concepts and ideas and why did some of us find it incredibly difficult? What was it that prevented us from learning the same things at the same time? As a result, how we learn has been a great source of interest for educational psychologists and educationalists for many years and, in an attempt at an explanation, they have developed numerous models of learning.

Each of these has a bearing on how effective your teaching is and a brief overview follows here. There are many excellent publications and websites available, if you wish to explore this area further; some of these are listed at the end of this chapter.

Research undertaken by Säljö (1979) found that what students understood by learning fell into five distinct categories.

1. Learning to acquire information, thus increasing knowledge

2. Learning to memory; for example, 'swotting up' for exams to be reproduced at the appropriate time

3. Learning for the 'as and when', which can be retained and used as necessary

4. Learning in the abstract: this requires the ability to apply subject matter to a different context or situation and to the real world

5. Learning as understanding reality in a different way, which requires us to understand what is happening around us by continually reinterpreting knowledge.

ACTIVITY 1.5

Take a few moments to reflect on how this applies to what we learn in order to carry out our current roles. You may have identified that all of the examples given have a bearing in some way. For example, some of the categories are quite straigt-forward in that learning is something that we acquire, whereas some involve a much more complex view, requiring us to be able to interpret the learning and apply it to different situations.

The above theory is about students' understanding of learning, whereas the theories that follow focus on *how* we learn.

Behaviourist

These theories are based on what is termed stimulus and response. This means that the student responds largely to a stimulus, that is, information provided by the teacher, rather than to any other forces. This implies that the student is relatively passive in the learning process, and learning is largely dependent on input from others. The emphasis is on 'conditioning' the student to respond in a given way to given situations.

Classical conditioning

Classical conditioning was first described by Pavlov (1927), who observed that dogs normally salivated at the sight of food. This he termed an unconditioned response, as it was inherent in the dog without any training being required. Pavlov then sounded a bell before the dog received its food, and discovered it was possible to train the dog to salivate to the ringing of the bell rather than to the production of food – a *conditioned* response.

Operant conditioning

This theory is also based on stimulus and response, but relies on a system of effective training by using rewards. The psychologist Skinner (1968) discovered that it was possible for pigeons to learn how to operate a lever to deliver their food; the food was both their reward and the factor that reinforced their learning of how to use the lever. He used a 'schedule of reinforcements' which had to be applied consistently. Further reading on behaviourism can be found at http://www.learning-theories.com/behaviorism.html.

You may ask how such theories can possibly help you, as a practitioner involved in teaching. This is not necessarily a wrong assumption. It has been identified by some that Skinner's generalisations concerning human behaviour reflect the study of animals which are totally unlike human beings. That said, supporters of classical conditioning reason that, although it acknowledges the need for refinement, Pavlov's work can be used to shape the intellectual development of students. This view, much simplified, is based on the fact that Pavlov demonstrated that learning is dependent on interaction with the contextual circumstances. For example, students may learn the type of behaviour expected of them in the classroom situation just by being there.

Cognitive or humanistic

These theories are more student-centred and, as a result, are much easier to apply in nursing. Cognition means the act of knowing (*Concise Oxford Dictionary* 1999), and involves students' own thinking and perception. The approach centres on the work of a psychologist named Karl Rogers. Rogers includes in the act of knowing the feelings of the student, and the need to recognise his or her individuality – the humanistic approach. For example, and very simplified, students learn best when they can relate to previous experiences and apply these to their current learning.

Social and situational learning

Social learning is based on the assumption that people learn from observing other people. When applied to nursing education it is an extremely useful tool as it allows people to see the outcomes and consequences of other's behaviour and, as a result, they are able to gain some understanding of the results of their action. This is further developed in Chapter 2.

DOMAINS OF LEARNING

Bloom (1972) has identified three areas, or domains, in which learning takes place and which provide a useful framework for the practitioner involved in teaching. These are:

1. The *cognitive* domain, concerned with the acquisition of knowledge

2. The *psychomotor* domain, relating to the development of skills. This in itself is a very useful domain for planning teaching and will be further developed in Chapter 2

3. The *affective* domain, involving attitude formation.

The cognitive domain is about how we acquire information, and what we need to know, as opposed to what we need to do. For example, this could be the effects of compression bandaging on a limb, or how insulin works.

The psychomotor domain involves the act of doing, or skills acquisition. This could be learning how to give an intramuscular injection, or how to record an electrocardiogram.

The affective domain relates to the development of beliefs, values and attitudes. An example of this is the acceptance of a patient's right to refuse consent to, or to comply with, specific treatment.

The following scenario will help in your understanding of the three domains.

Staff Nurse White is teaching compression bandaging to a group of students. First, she provides the students with knowledge of the circulatory system and how to identify a venous leg ulcer. This is learning in the cognitive domain.

Next, Staff Nurse White teaches them how to apply compression bandaging. This lies in the psychomotor domain.

Finally, she discusses with the students the patient's attitude to wearing compression bandaging and the need to ensure that it is accepted by the patient if treatment is to be effective. This is learning in the affective domain.

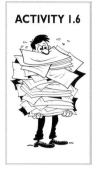

ACTIVITY 1.6

Identify a piece of teaching that you have recently undertaken. In which of the domains did learning take place?

It is essential to consider all three domains in our teaching, even though we may not always use them all. It is unlikely that any single theory or model will account for all aspects of learning that take place, but it appears that the cognitive theories previously outlined can help students to acquire problem-solving skills that they will require in their future roles. The stimulus–response or conditioning theories, with their emphasis on reinforcement, point to the importance of immediate feedback in the learning situation.

However useful models and theories may be in identifying how we learn, there are numerous other factors that are key to effective learning. In particular, we need to consider what issues are important for the adult learner, and how individual differences will affect the learning that takes place.

FACTORS INFLUENCING LEARNING

There are numerous factors that influence how we learn.

Learning and perception

In psychology, perception is the process of acquiring, interpreting, selecting and organising sensory information. That is, the information we acquire from what we see, speak, hear, smell or feel. As a result it is easy to see why, as individuals, what we perceive is so important to both the teaching and learning process and to patient/client care. There are many perceptual theories that tell us how we process thoughts and how our understanding affects learning, pariticularly how we store information in memory. The trick to storage, of course, is to be able to retrieve things as and when we need them and, probably more importantly, to be aware that we need to store the imformation in the first place!.

Whatever is being learned is dependent on how information is arranged in your student's mind. For example, when learning, students may screen some things out as irrelevant or not comprehensible. That is why checking understanding, asking questions and linking knowledge directly to your patients' experiences will help students classify information and underpin understanding that enables them to store the information in their long-term memory.

Sociological factors affecting learning

The most relevant sociological factors that may influence the learning process are those of language, social class and culture. These are not new to the body of knowledge about how people learn. As far back as 1962, Bernstein identified what he terms a 'restricted language code', which is closely linked to child-rearing practices and education. He argues that people from a working-class background use a limited vocabulary compared with the middle and upper classes, who have a much more elaborate language code. This ultimately affects the way in which people think and make sense of the world around them. If this view is accepted, it would obviously have a bearing on the learning process, as teachers and students would not necessarily be 'speaking the same language'.

Another important aspect of language is that of *meaning*. This is neatly summed up in the phrase 'I know you think you heard what I said, but what you heard is not what I meant!' Put another way, sometimes the words we use may have a different meaning for the person with whom we are communicating. The words of the hospital 'spokesperson' provide us with a perfect example of this: the patient's condition is usually described as 'comfortable' even if the patient is suffering from multiple fractures.

Culture, in its broadest sense, relates to the shared beliefs, values and understanding that are subscribed to by identifying with a particular group. Any student group will link into a culture or subculture of one type or another. For example, patients or clients, as a group, tend to identify with one another in terms of common problems, and we encourage this by introducing them to self-help groups. e.g. Diabetes UK or Mencap. The teacher needs to understand in patients the accepted values, attitudes and behaviours of the culture or subculture in order to establish a rapport with the student. Mead (1934) states that we all start off by learning roles from our parents and then complete our socialisation by internalising – that is, accepting as our own – the norms and values of other membership groups, at both the cultural and the subcultural levels. We also tend to become labelled by others according to the cultures and subcultures in which we find ourselves.

The cultural influences brought to bear on students are of enormous consequence, as they may be of far greater importance to the student than those imparted by the teacher. For example, for adolescents their relationship to their peer group is very important, and they would often rather please their peers than their family or teachers. As a result, much of what the teacher tries to achieve will be of no consequence if it is not accepted by the peer group.

As another example, if you were teaching health promotion to a group of students, you would need to estimate the influence of their peer group. If your session was on the effects of smoking, it would be easier to demonstrate the ill effects to a group whose peers did not smoke and whose original socialisation to non-smoking behaviour was because their parents did not smoke. It would obviously be harder to convince a group of the ill effects of smoking if their parents had always smoked and members of their peer group also smoked. Teachers must therefore be aware that culture can have a great bearing on the effectiveness of learning.

The importance of individual differences

As was identified earlier in the chapter, individual differences play a crucial role in how and what we learn. If this were not the case then teaching would be extremely easy, as all we would need to do is tell every student the information and it would all be readily understood at the same rate. Clearly, this is not the case.

Motivation

It is impossible to think about how we learn without thinking about why we want to do it! To say that a person must want to learn in order for learning to take place seems self-evident, but there are many factors (within both the teaching and the learning process) that will contribute to the student's wish to learn. Motivation is largely about the influences that drive an individual to achieving certain goals. These can be either internal or external: for example, the wish to improve one's knowledge or the wish to succeed in order to please someone else.

There are many definitions of motivation that can be found by entering the word into your search engine on the internet.

For example, what makes a student who has completed a diploma course move on to a degree? Or an overworked ward manager stay on the ward after his or her span of duty has finished?

Motivation can be described as either intrinsic or extrinsic to the individual. Intrinsic motivation relates to the personal factors that make us want to learn. The theorist Maslow (1987) provides a good example of intrinsic motivation. He identifies five levels of need that must be met for a person to reach his or her fullest potential:

1. *Physiological*: When applied to student learning, this means that if the student environment is, for example, over- or underheated, or noisy – or if the student is hungry or tired – learning is unlikely to take place, or may be limited.
2. *Safety*: Students need to feel safe from danger at every level. For example, students may feel 'unsafe' in an environment where they do not know other students, or do not have confidence in the teacher.
3. *Social*: This involves the 'need to be needed' (or valued) in both our home and our working life, for example to be accepted by our colleagues.
4. *Self-esteem*: When applied to student learning, self-esteem means the need for mutual respect between the individual student, the students as a group, and the teacher.
5. *Self-actualisation*: Maslow claims that it is only when these individual needs have been met that students are able to reach their full potential and have the opportunity to 'become everything one is capable of becoming' (Sargent 1990, p. 5).

There are, however, other intrinsic factors that will influence learning – for example, your personal feelings regarding your relationship with other students and teachers.

Extrinsic motivation is that which occurs outside the student, and over which he or she may have no control. It is important to note here that the two types of motivation are rarely exclusive of each other. For example, the way in which students are welcomed on to the ward or clinic will undoubtedly affect how they feel – no one likes to feel unwelcome!

ACTIVITY 1.7

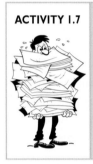

Think of a course of study you have recently undertaken. Try to identify the factors that made you want to learn. Were these intrinsic, extrinsic or a mixture of both? If the course of study you identified was in nursing, it is likely that you identified some of the extrinsic factors of motivation – for example the need to pass examinations in order to practise in a particular role or specialism. Indeed, your salary or promotion may depend on it.

As noted above, these two aspects are by no means exclusive of each other, as students of nursing normally enter education with a high degree of intrinsic motivation. This can then be overtaken by extrinsic factors, particularly the need to pass examinations.

LEARNING STYLES

What they are and what they mean

As can now be seen, the importance of getting to know students' individual characteristics and needs is crucial if learning is to be effective. This is largely a result of the individual's own learning style, sometimes referred to as *cognitive* style.

Research undertaken by psychologists has identified basic differences in our preferred way of learning. Put simply, it is argued that there are many different ways in which we approach and process information. For example, some students find the use of diagrams helpful when learning, whereas others prefer to rely solely on the written word. As a result there are many different views and thoughts relating to learning styles and some of them will be described below. In addition there are a number of excellent websites which will not only acquaint you with the many theorists but also provide you with self-assessment tools for finding out more about your individual learning styles. Two of these are www.businessballs .com/vaklearningstylestest.htm and www.studyskills.soton.ac.uk/studyguides/ Learning%20styles.doc.

Types of learning styles

The value of having an understanding of an individual's learning style is that it enables us to utilise learning methods and experiences that fit individual preferences and, as a result, enhance learning.

Honey and Mumford (cited in Stengelhofen 1996, pp. 54–55) identify four distinct learning styles that are useful in helping us to understand individual learning needs (Box 1.1). They state that students can be categorised into *activists*, *pragmatists*, *theorists* or *reflectors*.

ACTIVITY 1.8

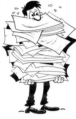

What characteristics do you think individuals would possess in each of the four categories? The names that have been given to the four categories provide us with a very good indication of the preferred learning style of the individual.

BOX 1.1	*Four categories of learning style*

Activists
- Like novelty
- Energetic
- Easily bored
- Open-minded
- Enjoy working alongside others
- Live for the present

Reflectors
- Like time to think
- Thorough
- Avoid reaching speedy conclusions
- Are observers as opposed to leaders

Theorists
- Analyse situations
- Systematic
- Have the ability to reason
- Need to know logic behind actions and observations

Pragmatists
- Learning dictated by practical consequences rather than theory
- Receptive to new ideas
- Like things to happen quickly

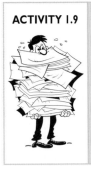

ACTIVITY 1.9 Think where your own learning style, or those of your students, may lie in relation to the four categories identified. Although Box 1.1 provides only a short description, it is clear that the teaching method we use could affect whether the student will learn new information. For example, a student who has an activist learning style may have difficulty learning from a lecture in which there is no student interaction. A reflector may find learning from role play problematic, as that would depend on an immediate response from the student. Varying your teaching methods will undoubtedly appeal to your students' different learning styles.

Visual, auditory and kinaesthetic learning styles

Having a visual learning style means, as the word implies, that it is what can be seen that enables and enhances learning. So, as an example, students with a visual learning style appreciate teaching that involves diagrams, pictures, handouts, films and demonstrations.

A student with an auditory learning style appreciates information that is transferred through listening, so the spoken word of self or others is important to learning.

Kinaesthetic learning is what is termed the 'act of doing'. Students learn best by being involved in 'hands-on' experiences and by touching, feeling and handling.

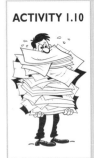

ACTIVITY 1.10 Take a few moments to reflect on your style in relation to the above theory. It is important to note that, although giving us an indication as to how we may learn best, these styles are not in themselves absolute. For example, I find it practically impossible to undertake serious reading when there is any form of background noise. Whilst this might indicate I do not have an auditory learning style, it does not necessarily mean I am unable to process anything via this route.

Experiential learning styles

Kolb (1984), building on the work of previous theorists, identified what he termed as an experiential learning styles model. It is a complex model that is based on a four-stage learning cycle and four resulting learning styles. In Kolb's model the student's experience (or what is currently happening to the student) enables the student to reflect, resulting in new ideas and potential outcomes. He describes this as a cycle of experiencing, reflecting, thinking and acting.

From this cycle Kolb was able to identify different learning styles which he subsequently termed diverging, assimilating, converging and accommodating:

- A *diverging* learning style draws on experience, reflecting on what has been observed. This gives students the ability to analyse tasks from a number of different viewpoints. Such students are 'ideas developers'.

- An *assimilating* learning style combines the ability to conceptualise abstract ideas and reflective observation. Generally, such people are good problem-solvers and are able to sort and categorise information from a variety of sources. They tend to be very structured in their thinking.

- *Converging* learning styles are demonstrable in students who combine experimentation and abstract concepts. Such students are particularly good at learning from experience and applying what has been learned to future scenarios.

- *Accommodating* learning styles have their basis in concrete experience and being able to experiment. These students, according to Kolb, are not necessarily logical but demonstrate a practical approach to problem-solving.

LEARNING THROUGH MEDIATION CHANNELS

Gregorc's theory (1982) is based on the notion that there are two distinct channels through which we receive and then express information. He termed these mediation channels *perceptions* and *ordering*. They are closely linked to the section on perception described earlier in the chapter.

Gregorc identifies two types of individuals under the perceptions channel: those who prefer to deal with what is (i.e. the concrete world) and those who prefer to deal with concepts and feelings.

In describing the *ordering* channel Gregorc identifies students who like to organise their learning in a step-by-step manner as opposed to others who prefer to organise their learning randomly.

LOCUS OF CONTROL

That which could be seen to be quite contradictory to the learning styles identified above is the view of the importance of a locus of control that ultimately influences how we learn. The theory is based on work undertaken by Rotter (1966) which relates to how individual attitudes and beliefs affect the ways in which we live. The theory again relates clearly to perception as it is largely about whether or not, as individuals, we perceive that what we achieve in life, for example on a personal level happy relationships, or on a work level promotion, is brought about either by ourselves (internal locus of control) or by forces that are outside our control (external locus of control). A clear and full description of Rotter's theory can be found at www.psych.fullerton.edu/jmearns/rotter.htm.

Again, it is important to note here that an internal and external locus of control is not absolute and is best viewed as a continuum. Most individuals would not perceive everything that happens in their life to be either totally within or outside their control, although I am sure we all know people who hold the view of passive victim in that 'it always happens to me'.

Whilst the above theories go some way to identifying the complexities of how we learn, the nature of this chapter does not allow for an indepth analysis of their respective strengths and weaknesses. Further and much more detailed information can be found by accessing the references provided at the end of this chapter.

WAYS OF LEARNING

In addition to paying attention to the different styles of learning when teaching, there are also many different ways in which we learn that we can utilise to make teaching more effective. Here are just some of them. Some aspects, particularly reflection, will be developed further in Chapter 4 and as a result this is only dealt with briefly here.

Learning by reflection

You will already have identified from your experiences of CPD the value of reflective practice, both to the teacher and to the whole of the learning process. The principles of this are particularly relevant to this chapter in terms of enhancing the learning experience for the student.

Reflection is about analysing a situation in order to decide on the best way forward and to learn from it. Boud et al (1985) identify a preparatory phase in the reflective process in which the student consciously anticipates the experience. It is argued that this is an essential part of learning and that its value should not be overlooked. In view of this, reflection is concerned with looking forward to experiences as well as learning from what has passed.

There are four key points that are crucial to becoming proficient in the process of reflective practice:

1. The need for conscious and voluntary effort

2. Its usefulness as a tool in helping you to explore the links between what you are told and your observations in practice

3. The importance of journal-writing in assisting the reflective process

4. The need to work through initial difficulties in journal-writing as these diminish with persistence and practice.

Sitting by Nellie

The term sitting by, or next to, Nellie, is used to describe on-the-job training by existing members of staff. It arguably has its origins in the industrial north when people learned how to work the woollen and cotton looms by observing the person next to them. There are advantages and disadvantages to this method of learning, although used in the right way it is a very powerful learning tool.

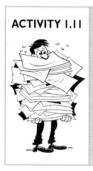

ACTIVITY 1.11

Can you identify the advantages and disadvantages for students learning in this way? An advantage is that the student will learn well if the person acting as Nellie has all the right ingredients, for example, the appropriate knowledge, skills, expertise and motivation. When this is the case there can be no better way of learning. I am sure almost all of us can identify a great role model from our past. On the other hand, if the person acting as Nellie is not sufficiently skilled or motivated then the results can be disastrous.

As a practitioner teaching students you need to be aware of both of these aspects.

Participative learning

As can be seen from the learning styles already identified, actively participating in a learning activity can greatly enhance a student's capacity to retain knowledge and ideas. In addition, active participation can also help students to learn much more than specific facts. For example, students actively taking part in a debate are exposed to many other factors which help them to develop different skills and aptitudes, such as:

- Learning to listen to others
- Learning to respond quickly
- Gaining confidence in public speaking
- Learning how to organise their thoughts
- Putting forward a cohesive argument.

Enquiry-based learning (EBL)

EBL fits neatly into the model of andragogy discussed earlier, as it is a process that is largely student-owned. It usually follows a given format:

1. Students are given a specific scenario, for example, support available for people who are visually impaired.

2. Students are then required to undertake an examination of the resources they will need to research that will provide them with the appropriate information.

3. From this, students are able to generate their own issues and questions.

ACTIVITY 1.12

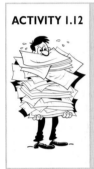

What are the benefits of this type of learning?
You may have identified some of the following in your answer:

- It enables students to take responsibility for their own learning
- It enables students to identify where their individual gaps in knowledge are
- It can further develop their research according to their own interests
- It encourages team-working.

Problem-based learning (PBL)

PBL does effectively 'what it says on the tin'. It starts from a problem, specific question or indeed a scenario, as identified above. Students usually work together in groups supported by a facilitator. Students then share their existing knowledge relating to the scenario with the rest of the group, jointly agree what it is they need to learn and the resources they will require in order to do it. Once identified, students undertake this work, reconvening frequently to discuss and evaluate their work and also agree the next steps in the process.

The differences between EBL and PBL are not immediately obvious and they have been the subject of much debate within education since they emerged as a valuable learning tool. Generally, EBL can be seen as the umbrella term that incorporates PBL, whereas PBL itself is much more specific, utilising scenarios that have been specifically designed for the purpose.

Work-based learning

Work-based learning is learning that is primarily focused in the workplace, although it is often supported by theoretical learning as part of a structured course or programme. Increasingly it is becoming a very effective method for healthcare professionals, for example nurses, doctors and allied health professionals working and learning together in the practice environment.

Lifelong learning

If you were to search the term 'lifelong learning' on the internet you would make at least one million 'hits'. This is because, although not a new concept, lifelong learning has been high on the agendas of the government, education providers, employers, employees and students since the publication of the government's Green Paper *The Learning Age* (accessible at www.life-longlearning.co.uk/greenpaper/ch-fore.htm). Lifelong learning is based on the belief that a culture of lifelong learning is needed by society in order to develop an inclusive society in which all individuals are valued and are able to achieve their maximum potential. It is believed that, in so doing, a society that is able to prosper in an increasingly competitive world can be secured. It is based on the need for us all as individuals to take responsibility for our own development, which in turn will lead to a society which has learning at its heart. As a government-supported issue it is very similar in principle to developments in healthcare which focus on patient/client involvement and the development of systems and processes to enable patients to take responsibility for their own health.

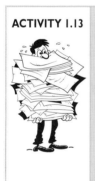

ACTIVITY 1.13

Take a few moments to think about the term 'lifelong learning' and consider what this means for you in your professional life. You may choose to explore the definition by accessing some of the million hits mentioned above but your own view is equally relevant here.

You may have identified issues such as learning in a formal and structured way as opposed to the types of learning we gain just by being and the constant development of your knowledge and how this will influence your practice.

In addition, you may have identified some clear links between lifelong learning and the need for continuing professional development.

This is explored in more detail in the following section.

Continuing professional development

As with lifelong learning, there are many different definitions put forward by organisations to describe CPD, but all definitions include the need for enhancing knowledge, expertise and competence as part of a lifelong learning process.

It is important to note that, whilst CPD is important to us as practising nurses, it is equally important to our employers in that it is crucial to their developing the workforce they require to meet future healthcare need.

It is also crucial to patient safety and quality standards of patient/client care and is the raison d'être of the Nursing and Midwifery Council (NMC) – the governing body of nurses, midwives and community specialist public health nurses.

ACTIVITY 1.14

What do you think are the benefits of CPD to yourself, your employer and your patients and clients?

You will no doubt have identifed some of the following:

- For yourself: personal ambition to be a better practitioner, improving your career options, increasing levels of confidence, increasing your professional status, improving your financial income, gaining higher qualifications, a requirement by the NMC to maintain your professional status.
- For your employer: to ensure that nurses in the future are able to meet future healthcare need, for example, as in the current initiatives to provide care to patients closer to home, to ensure competence to ensure safety and to provide a framework for pay.
- For your patients/clients: all patients have a right to expect practitioners to be able to provide safe and competent care based on up-to-date knowledge and research.

There are six underlying principles of CPD:

1. It is necessary to ensure patient safety and enhance and improve patient care.

2. CPD exemplifies the wish of the individual to improve performance continually.

3. The responsibility for CPD is owned by the individual practitioner.

4. CPD must take account of individual learning needs, career planning and the needs of the employer. (This is usually brought together through the annual appraisal.)

5. Outcomes should be clearly defined and measurable.

6. Investment in terms of both time and funding is crucial to effective CPD.

As you will already be aware, nurses, midwives and health visitors meet their CPD requirements following registration through Post-Registration Education and Practice (PREP), administered by the NMC. Its purpose is to improve the standards of patient and client care. The NMC requires all nurses, midwives and health visitors to meet both a CPD standard which identifies the ongoing educational requirements of PREP, and a practice standard which determines the practice requirements for PREP.

The PREP (CPD) standard

This standard requires that you undertake a minimum of 35 hours of learning activity during the 3-year period between the dates of your registration renewal. It is important to note that learning activity implies not solely formal learning, e.g. study days, but also private study and learning from others.

The PREP (Practice) standard

Since 1995 the PREP (Practice) Standard has required you to have been 'working in some capacity by virtue of a qualification in nursing, midwifery or community specialist public health nurse for not less than 100 days or 750 hours during the 5 years before renewal of your registration'. This standard was revised in 2006 and with effect from 1 August 2006 the timescale was brought into line with the PREP (CPD) standard, i.e. over a 3-year period. This means that the practice standard is now 450 hours over 3 years.

Detailed information on the process and your responsibilities regarding PREP can be found in the NMC PREP handbook on the NMC website at www.nmc-uk.org/aDisplayDocument.aspx?DocumentID=1636.

LEARNING ENVIRONMENTS

The surroundings in which students learn can greatly influence their ability to learn and are therefore of importance when planning teaching. Some of these issues are further developed in the next chapter. A learning environment however is much more than the physical surroundings students experience. How, or indeed whether, a student learns can also be greatly influenced by his or her employer's views and commitment to learning (are they a learning organisation?) and equally whether they have an established culture of learning throughout the organisation.

Creating learning organisations and learning cultures

As can be seen from the previous section, if lifelong learning is to be at the heart of society then it is crucial that organisations view learning as central to the way in which they deliver their business. Handy (1999) describes organisations as needing to demonstrate the E factor – excitement, enthusiasm, effervescence and energy – and believes that 'organisations learn only through individuals who learn. Individual learning does not guarantee organisational learning. But without it no organisational learning occurs' (Handy 1999).

A learning organisation therefore allows staff to learn and grow both personally and professionally.

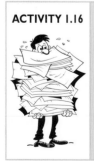

ACTIVITY 1.15   Based on Handy's views above, what factors do you think would lead you to believe that you were part of a learning organisation?

   You may have identified some of the following:

- There is visible leadership
- Staff are encouraged to discuss and exchange ideas
- Training needs are met and evaluated
- There are clear appraisal systems
- Facilities are available for learning, e.g. books, internet access
- Staff development systems are apparent at practice level.

The culture of an organisation 'or indeed a workplace' is central to effective learning as it is largely through this that behaviour, whether negative or positive, is learned. The culture is crucial to the way we are socialised into work and is extremely important when new staff, particularly students, become part of the working team. Socialisation is the process by which people become part of a culture and is the process by which we learn how different groups work. It is an extremely important concept for a learning organisation where colleagues can effectively be socialised into the values and beliefs that underpin the organisation. In recent years this has been taken much more seriously by healthcare employers, as they regularly undertake and publish the results of surveys to assess employees' views on the organisation as being a 'good' employer.

Staff surveys can be a very useful tool in establishing whether staff within an organisation are motivated and as a result performing to best effect.

As a teacher, the level to which you are inspirational, motivational and persuasive are key to how you can effectively persuade and motivate others. As most of us will know from personal experience, when we feel fairly or advantageously treated we are more likely to be motivated. When we feel unfairly treated, we are much more likely to feel isolated, powerless and uninvolved which, in turn, is a serious demotivator.

ACTIVITY 1.16

Take a few minutes to consider your own practice setting. What kind of culture does it exhibit? Is it supportive? Does it encourage communication and new ideas? Is it welcoming to new members of staff and students?

   In an ideal situation the above characteristics would be present but if they are not the following will help you to develop them.

Creating a learning environment for your students

There are positive steps that can be taken to create a learning environment for your student within the practice setting. Hart and Rotem (1995) identify six factors which are fundamental to an effective learning environment. Each one holds a strong message for us all as teachers and ensuring they are present demonstrates that there are tangible things that can be done to change and/or improve it.

- *Autonomy and recognition*: The extent to which staff are valued, acknowledged and encouraged to take responsibility for their own practice
- *Job satisfaction*: The extent to which nurses enjoy their work and intend to pursue a career in nursing
- *Role clarity*: The extent to which staff understand and accept their role and responsibilities
- *Quality of supervision*: The extent to which supervision and staff interaction facilitate or impede improved practice
- *Peer support*: The extent to which staff are friendly, caring and supportive of one another
- *Opportunities for learning*: The extent to which learning opportunities are restricted or available.

Remember that any changes needed in the above can start with you! Frequently it only takes one leading light to initiate change!

EVALUATING LEARNING

Evaluation is extremely important throughout all aspects of healthcare in order to ensure both the effectiveness and value of what we are doing. It is particularly important in education as it is one of the primary means of knowing what has been learned (and ultimately what will change as a result of it). The process of evaluation is dealt with in much greater depth in Chapter 2 but there are some key purposes of evaluation that are relevant to the learning process in that they:

- provide information for stakeholders
- help to ensure that objectives are met
- identify staff training and development needs
- identify problems and weakness so they can be corrected
- provide information to assist future development

It is important to note that the evaluation process is likely to be driven by many different factors, for example, the curriculum (as in pre-registration education programmes) and the requirements of validation bodies such as the NMC.

CONCLUSION

This chapter has focused on factors that have a bearing on the ways in which we learn, and how we can maximise learning in our own working environment.

Just as human behaviour is extremely complex, so too is the learning theory that underpins it. As a result the purpose of this chapter has been to provide you in a straightforward way with some of the building blocks on which to base your teaching. The fact that learning and teaching are so closely linked will also influence the way in which we teach, in either the classroom or the practice setting, and this is developed in Chapter 2.

REFERENCES

Bernstein B (1962) Linguistic codes, hesitation phenomina and intelligence. Language and Speech 5: 15–17

Bloom B S (1972) Taxonomy of educational objectives. London: Longman

Boud D, Keogh R, Walker D (1985) Reflections: turning experience into learning. London: Kogan Page

Concise Oxford Dictionary, 10th edn (1999) United States: Oxford University Press.

Gregorc A (1982) An adult's guide to style. Columbia, CT: Gregorc Associates

Handy C (1999) Inside organizations: 21 ideas for managers. London: Penguin Books

Hart G, Rotem A (1995) The clinical learning environment: nurses' perceptions of professional development in clinical settings. Nurse Education Today 15: 3–10

Kolb D (1984) Experiential learning. New York: Prentice Hall

Maslow A H (1987) Motivation and personality. London: Harper and Row

Mead G H (1934) Mind, self and society. Chicago: University of Chicago Press

Osler W (1989) In: Daintith J, Isaacs A. Medical quotations. Collins reference dictionary. Glasgow: Market House Books, P. 200

Pavlov I P (1927) Classics in the history of psychology. Cited at www.psychclassics. yorku.ca/Pavlov

Quinn F M, Hughes S J (2007) Quinn's principles and practice of nurse education, 5th edn. Cheltenham: Nelson Thornes

Rotter J (1966) Generalised expectations for internal versus external control of reinforcement. Psychological Monographs 80: 1

Säljö R (1979) Cited at http://www.users. globalnet.co.uk/~infed/ohps/exhibits/saljo_ learning.htm

Sargent A (1990) Turning people on: the motivation challenge. London: Institute of Personnel Management

Skinner B F (1968) The technology of teaching. New York: Appleton-Century-Croft

Stengelhofen J (1996) Teaching students in clinical settings. London: Chapman & Hall

2 How to make your teaching effective

Sue Howard

INTRODUCTION

As readers of this book you will be teaching for different reasons and to achieve different things. For example, some of you will be teaching as part of a set and detailed curriculum, such as a pre-registration nursing programme, whilst others may just want some tips on how best to help students understand how to undertake a specific skill or task, or to make a presentation.

Even the most confident and competent of teachers will admit to a degree of nervousness when asked to undertake a presentation for the first time, but with the right approach and preparation this can become a very enjoyable part of the practitioner's role. The purpose of this part of the chapter is, therefore, to provide you with the 'how to' of teaching by giving you a framework within which to make your teaching effective. It will identify strategies that you can employ in order to maximise your students' learning and enable you to plan, execute and evaluate your teaching appropriately.

LEARNING OBJECTIVES

After reading this chapter you should be able to:

◆ Identify, discuss and adopt some of the teaching strategies that will make your teaching effective

◆ Identify and discuss some major structures and processes within which nurse teaching is based

◆ Utilise a variety of teaching methods in your teaching

◆ Understand the importance of evaluating your teaching

◆ Identify and discuss some methods that can be used to evaluate your teaching successfully.

TEACHING STRATEGIES

In Chapter 1 we explored the issues that can have a strong influence on how students learn and what may help or hinder their learning. Much in the same way there are some strategies we can adopt that will maximise the chance of our teaching being effective.

Building the framework: why we need a teaching strategy

A strategy, in its simplest form, is concerned with forward planning. The *Concise Oxford Dictionary* (1999) describes it as 'the art of war; especially the part of it concerned with the conduct of campaigns'. This may appear to be a rather extreme definition, but those of you who have had the experience of teaching a group of over 200 pre-registration nursing students are unlikely to deny the need to be organised.

Some years ago, as a nurse relatively new to classroom teaching, I came across research that suggested that there was little correlation between well-prepared teaching and the students' ability to learn. I tried it with a new group of post-registration students undertaking a module on coronary heart disease. I don't recommend it! Preparation is the key. As a general rule, if you know that you are unprepared for what it is you are going to teach, then your students will too.

TEACHING A SKILL

Teaching skills is probably the most important aspect of the role of practitioners, either in teaching patients/clients to undertake a particular procedure for themselves or teaching student nurses skills, such as the safe moving and handling of patients.

As experienced practitioners, many of the skills that you undertake in your daily work, for example the positioning of your feet prior to moving a patient, are largely carried out subconsciously. It is likely that, because of the amount of practice you have had at performing the procedure, it has become instinctive or internalised.

We have learned from Chapter 1 that learning is enhanced if the material is provided in a logical sequence. This is particularly relevant when teaching a skill, as the action can be broken down into a series of stages or steps.

Teaching a skill involves learning in both the cognitive and the motor domains (see Chapter 1).

If skills can be broken down into a series of steps they are much more easily understood, although there are other factors for us to consider, for example the level of motivation of the student and how the subject is presented by the teacher.

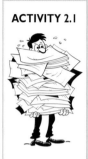

ACTIVITY 2.1

Imagine that you have a new student nurse on your ward and you want to teach her how to administer a drug safely to a patient. Write down the steps you would need to go through in order to complete the task.

You will want to check the following items, although their order may change depending on your individual preference:

- The name of the drug against the patient's drug administration record
- The dosage of the drug
- The time the drug is to be given
- That it is being given to the correct patient by asking the patient
- That the name on the patient's armband confirms this
- That the patient does not have any known allergies to the drug about to be given
- That the administration of the drug has been accurately recorded.

Preparing your teaching

One of the greatest difficulties for most practitioners faced with teaching for the first time is where to start. As identified in Chapter 1, it is clear that the teaching method you select can affect the way in which students learn, so an assessment of your student or student group is essential.

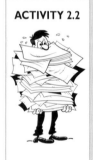

ACTIVITY 2.2

Think about the types of experience that are available in your area of work, what aspects you could teach to students and what method would be most effective. Of course this will differ greatly depending on whether you work in the hospital or community or acute or critical care.

Whatever your area of work your answer will undoubtedly reflect your personal learning style. There is, however, a sequence of events that can be applied regardless of the method selected. There is an old adage that is well known to teachers:

Tell 'em what you're going to tell 'em.
Then tell 'em.
Then tell 'em what you've just told 'em!

This principle can be applied to other situations. Next time you have the opportunity to view one of the old Hollywood slapstick comedies with the 'custard pie in the face' routine, watch carefully the sequence of events:

1. The deliverer of the custard pie indicates what is going to happen, i.e. he is going to let the receiver have it in the face! (Tell 'em what you're going to tell 'em.)

2. The deliverer delivers said custard pie to the recipient. (Then tell 'em.)

3. The deliverer holds empty plate, indicates the content on receiver's face and laughs. (Tell 'em what you've just told 'em!)

The sequence of events when planning teaching is therefore:

1. The introduction
2. The progression of the subject material
3. The conclusion.

The introduction includes 'setting the scene' for the session, finding out what the students already know, and telling them why they need to gain the knowledge and the method by which they are to learn it. Equally as important, regardless of the teaching method you choose, is the way in which you communicate with your students.

Communicating your teaching

As identified in Chapter 1, recent years have seen dramatic changes in the way we are taught and indeed how our learning is assessed. The movement has been from a 'chalk and talk' (pedagogical model) to an approach that is largely student-centred and student-led (andragogical model). For further information on these two approaches, please see page 4 in Chapter 1. Fundamental to this approach is the way in which we communicate our teaching material.

Here are some general rules to follow, both in preparation and during your teaching:

- Ask open as opposed to closed questions, for example:
    - What do you understand by that?
    - How would you do this?
    - What other view might you consider?

- Show an understanding of other people's feelings. You may be nervous teaching, but the student may also be afraid to speak.

- Listen carefully to what a student has to say.

Silence is possibly one of the most difficult situations to deal with when teaching, and 20 seconds' silence when you have posed a question does seem a really long time. This makes you vulnerable to answering your own questions rather than waiting for the student's response.

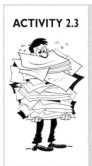

ACTIVITY 2.3

Position yourself as if you were speaking at the front of the class and ask a question (it doesn't matter what). Now wait 20 seconds. You will soon learn how long this can feel.

Give students alternatives. There is often more than one way of achieving the same goal.

Make sure that your facts are correct.

Do not be afraid of saying that you do not have an answer. Teachers never could, nor should they, know everything, but always say you'll find out – and do this!

Admit it openly if you get something wrong.

The use of humour in teaching

When used properly, humour is one of the most important qualities of a good teacher. The only major rules regarding the use of humour in your teaching are that its use should be appropriate and linked closely with the content of your teaching and also that it should never involve sarcasm or personal comments.

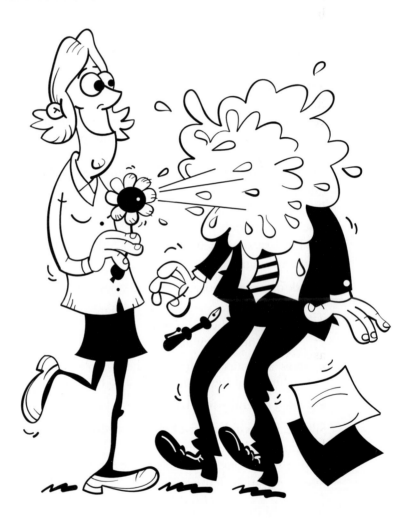

The importance of making your teaching evidence-based

Evidence-based practice can be described as the bridge between research and practice. As something we carry out, evidence-based practice is about the 'search, review and application of scientific evidence to the treatment and management of healthcare' (Hammer and Collinson 2005).

It is therefore incumbent on teachers to ensure that their teaching materials are from the same evidence-base. This can be achieved by always ensuring that you research your subject fully, and by providing the students with the evidence to support your statements and views.

One of the key purposes of evidence-based practice is to ensure that the patient/client receives up-to-date care based on up-to-date knowledge. It is therefore vital to the learning process that your information is not based on 'history'. The easiest way of ensuring this is by undertaking a literature search on the subject you are intending to teach. Your College of Nursing library will be able to assist you in this. It is important that your search is highly focused on what you want to know. For example, if you entered the words 'nursing process' you would get over 1000 'hits', which is obviously not much help. By asking yourself what exactly it is that you wish to know about the nursing process, you will narrow the subject down drastically and the information you receive will be much more manageable and pertinent. If you are not confident about this then do seek help from a faculty librarian.

THE WHAT, WHY, WHEN, WHERE AND HOW OF TEACHING

Having looked at some of the general issues, the following is a basic, but nonetheless useful, framework to use that will help you to feel more confident. It is often termed the 'what, why, when, where and how of teaching'.

The what of teaching

This aspect is not always quite as straightforward as it sounds, and many practitioners make the mistake of overlooking it. For example, you may be asked to deliver a teaching session on the moving and handling of patients, but what aspects of moving and handling are you required to teach? In reality, this can encompass legislation, aids to assist moving and handling, patient safety, nurse safety and employer policy. The possibilities are almost endless. This lesson was brought home to me very early in my teaching career when I was asked to deliver 10 hours' teaching on the learning environment!

Using the following as a guide will assist you in deciding exactly what you want the students to learn:

First, seek a clear answer to the fundamental question of what part of the subject you are being asked to teach. This will not only reduce your stress levels, but also enable you to focus your teaching and ensure that you are not repeating content that has already been taught.

Having identified the subject matter (you may sometimes have to be quite persistent about this), you are then in a position to develop the aim and specific objectives for the session (see below). Although it is acknowledged that the formulation of objectives may not always be the best way to plan your teaching, if you are new to teaching it does enable you to be much more focused. This is developed further in the next section.

The why of teaching

In order for you to gain an understanding of what is required in terms of teaching, it is essential to know *why* a particular subject is to be taught. For example:

- Is the subject an examinable part of the curriculum?
- If this is the case, what aspects of the subject must the students know?
- Does it link with previously taught subjects?

The when of teaching

There are five fundamental questions that you may find useful:

1. How much time have you been allocated for the session?
2. Is the time sufficient for what you have been asked to do?
3. How does what you have been asked to teach fit into the module or course? For example, is it a 'standalone' session or one of a series?
4. If others are teaching on the same subject, how can you ensure that there is no undue overlap or repetition? (Sometimes repetition can be helpful however.)
5. How will your teaching and the students' learning be evaluated?

The where of teaching

This may appear self-explanatory, but the changing numbers of student groups and the frequent, limited use of classroom accommodation often lead to various annexed buildings being used. It may be that your teaching is to take place in the practice area. If so, you will need to consider exactly where to carry out the teaching in order to avoid any distractions.

The how of teaching

Having gained the above information and established your objectives, you are now in a position to decide what is the most appropriate teaching method for the subject material you are to deliver.

PRACTICAL STEPS TO EFFECTIVE TEACHING

There are 10 practical steps you can take to make sure your teaching is effective and they all involve preparation. You cannot get away from it. If you want a good evaluation from students and clear evidence that learning has taken place you must think about what you want to achieve and how.

Providing a structure for your teaching

As practitioners there are very few things that we do as part of a working day that do not have structure, e.g. ward routines, mealtimes and administering medicines. Teaching is no different and is undoubtedly more effective when properly structured and planned.

Aims and objectives

Whether your teaching is to be formal (part of a curriculum) or a 'one-off', the development of aims and objectives as a framework for a planned teaching session is extremely useful. First, they provide a logical sequence for both you and your student, and second, they enable you to check whether your teaching has been effective. Central to the development of aims and objectives is the decision about what exactly the student should learn.

Identifying what to teach

This is often described as the must, should and could of teaching, and although it is a simple framework it will provide you with some very useful pegs on which to hang your subject material.

ACTIVITY 2.4

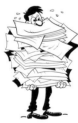

Think of a subject of which you have a sound knowledge. Here are some examples to help with your choice:

- Moving and handling of patients
- Storing drugs safely
- Planning off-duty rotas
- Care of a patient immediately following surgery.

Then, think about what it is about the subject that you feel the student *must* know, *should* know or *could* know in order to practise safely.

To take the safe storage of drugs as an example, you may feel that the students *must know* the following:

- The law relating to drug storage
- Your employer's policy on storage
- The process of recording stored drugs.

What they *should know* – that is, desirable additions to the must-knows – are the wider issues involved, for example the ordering and disposal of stored drugs.

Finally, what the students *could know* is non-essential but optional knowledge – for example, what is the patient's/client's role in storage?

This can provide a useful framework for identifying what is the most important content of your teaching and so should enable you to formulate your aim.

Identifying your aim for the session

An aim in teaching terms is an overall statement that identifies what the student must be able to do at the end of a given period of instruction or experience.

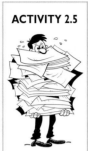

ACTIVITY 2.5

With this definition in mind, try to formulate an aim for the subject that you identified in Activity 2.4.

There are two key aspects to remember when identifying your aim: first, it is a general statement of what is to be achieved; and second, it should state why it is worth achieving.

To use the example of the care of a patient immediately following surgery, the aim for the teaching would be something like: 'At the end of the session, students will understand the key principles that underpin the care of a patient immediately following surgery, so that they can deliver skilled nursing care'. You will notice that the aim does not tell you how this will be achieved. This is done in the next step, by formulating educational objectives or what are now often called (intended) learning objectives.

Generally, objectives or learning outcomes must:

- Be achievable within the period allocated for the teaching
- Be specific in terms of what you want the student to achieve
- Be measurable in terms of their outcome.

Again, to use the care of a patient immediately following surgery as an example, the educational objectives could be as follows:

At the end of the session students should be able to:

- Explain the importance of maintaining a clear airway
- Recognise the signs and symptoms of an obstructed airway
- Describe the observations required on a patient immediately following surgery
- Recognise the factors that would require immediate medical assistance.

As a general rule by which to measure your objectives or learning outcomes, always ask whether they are SMART:

Specific

Measurable

Achievable

Realistic

Time-limited.

Useful as SMART objectives are in helping you to decide what to teach, they do have certain limitations.

| ACTIVITY 2.6 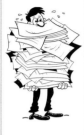 | Make a list of all the positive and negative aspects of teaching by objectives that you can think of. The positive aspects may include that they: |

- Provide your teaching with a clear and logical structure
- Enable the teacher to control the timing
- Make it easier to ascertain what the student has learned
- Provide a clear record of what has been taught
- Enable students to direct their own study.

The negative aspects may include that they:

- Are time-consuming to prepare (although this improves with practice)
- Tend to be inflexible
- Limit the content of the session and, as a result, what the student will learn.
- On balance, if you are new to teaching, using objectives when preparing to teach is invaluable.

Formal and informal teaching

Teaching is often described as being either informal or formal. Formal refers to the type of teaching that is preplanned, often with a clear aim and objectives. Informal teaching refers to the spontaneous type of teaching that occurs when a situation presents itself. Formal learning may include areas such as the safe moving and handling of patients or the care of essential equipment. Informal teaching could include the changing of intravenous fluids, which the student can observe at the bedside. Both these types of teaching have advantages for student learning.

The major advantage of using a formal method is that usually both the student and the teacher know exactly what the session aims to achieve. Further, the formal method enables the student to undertake his or her own preparation, for example by selecting some background reading. The major advantage of using an informal method is that it is meaningful for the student and helps to ensure that the knowledge he or she is gaining is up-to-date. This is often referred to as a form of 'action' learning.

Teaching part of a curriculum

Clearly, nurse education programmes need to be relevant to the area of work that students will be expected to undertake on completion of the course. Using pre-registration nurse education as an example, this is achieved through two elements:

1. The Nursing and Midwifery Council (NMC) sets the standards of proficiency required for pre-registration education and identifies the

core competencies that a nurse requires at the point of registration (NMC 2004).

2. The universities providing pre-registration programmes are responsible for curriculum planning, and the selection of an appropriate curriculum model with which to design the course that is able to demonstrate the standards set by the NMC.

3. The NMC gains assurance that the curriculum is meeting its set standards by ensuring that validation/visits take place at regular intervals. It is on this basis that universities receive approval to run the courses.

Use of curriculum models and their relevance to your teaching

Many of you will already be familiar with using nursing models to plan and prioritise care. In the same way, formalised programmes of nurse education are based on curriculum models. A curriculum model is basically a system for setting out the key elements of what should be learned and can be either in the form of the written word or diagrammatic. In nursing education it tends to be a mixture of both.

This section will provide you with a brief introduction to curriculum models, but for those who require a more in-depth knowledge, an excellent outline of curriculum planning and curriculum design is given by Quinn and Hughes (2007).

There are different models of curriculum design. The *product model* of curriculum design is based on the end result of education (usually an award or qualification) and the need to meet specific objectives. As identified in Chapter 1, learning is seen as a change in observable behaviour and is measured against the students' achievement of the objectives.

The *process model* of curriculum design depicts learning as intrinsically beneficial, rather than in terms of outcomes. Students are allowed to develop at their own pace, there are no set objectives, and as a result what is learned may be unpredictable.

The use of a product model in some aspects of nurse teaching can be extremely useful, especially when the completion of an end product of learning is required – for example, the teaching of fire evacuation procedures to a new student on the ward.

The process model is much more focused on the development of understanding, and so requires a more active role from students. It allows them to develop the skills they need at their own pace. In this model the teacher acts as a facilitator, supporting rather than telling the student what to do. There are no set outcomes to achieve by a given time – for example, the student learns over time how to prioritise care.

As a practitioner, facilitator or teacher, it is important that you are familiar with the curriculum design of the course with which you are involved if your teaching is to be effective, so don't be afraid to ask!

The following is a useful list of questions to ask when talking about this with a teacher or practitioner already involved in the development and implementation of the curriculum:

- What is the philosophy on which the curriculum is based?
- Which curriculum model has been chosen, and why?
- How do the different parts fit together to provide an overall package, for example, how are the students able to relate theory to practice and vice versa?
- How is progression demonstrated throughout the curriculum?
- Does the curriculum allow for differences in learning style?
- Does the curriculum allow for different teaching methods?
- How is the curriculum assessed?
- Does the model allow students to take responsibility for their own learning?

Creating an environment for teaching

The environment is wherever students are taught. However, it is well recognised from student feedback that the clinical situation is a particularly rich environment for teaching and learning, in that students' motivation to learn is high during their practical experience. This would seem to confirm that the place where students are most likely to be receptive to teaching and learning is the practice setting. This, in turn, makes it important that practitioners involved in teaching know how to create an environment conducive to learning.

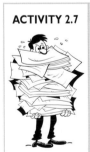

ACTIVITY 2.7

What key elements do you think are essential in creating a good environment for your students? To what extent do they exist in your own working environment? If they do not, how can you foster them?

You may have identified the need to be:

- Approachable
- Welcoming
- Confident enough in your work to pass information on to others
- Supportive
- Helpful
- Available and contactable
- Knowledgeable.

It is obvious that the more comfortable and safe we feel with the environment, the more likely it is that effective learning will take place.

Some of the aspects you have included in your answer will be developed further below.

TEACHING METHODS

Having identified what it is that you are going to teach and the environment in which you are going to teach it, you are then in a position to select an appropriate teaching method. There are many different methods that you can use, each of which has its advantages and disadvantages. However, the method selected needs to correspond to the domain of learning in which it is to take place if the learning is to be effective. A lecture is of little value if you wish to change students' attitudes on a given subject – for example, it is highly unlikely that you would change a student's opinion that inequalities in healthcare were justifiable by just lecturing to him or her.

Similarly, if we apply the model as set out by Maslow in Chapter 1, it is also necessary to consider the needs of the students. For example, learning is unlikely to take place if students are tired, hungry or any other of their basic needs have not been met.

The method chosen will also depend on the number of students you are going to teach, and there may be occasions when, because of the large number of students involved, a lecture is the only appropriate method. There is a variety of teaching methods that you can use:

- Lectures
- Group discussions
- Seminars
- Role-play
- Learning from critical incidents
- Independent/directed learning
- Experiential learning.

Problem-focused

The terms 'lecture' and 'lesson' are frequently used interchangeably, although a lesson tends to imply more student interaction. The lecture largely involves the teacher doing most of the talking, with the students listening. This can be an extremely good teaching method when you wish to provide the students with particular knowledge – for example the functions of the liver, or the results of certain research.

The lecture is extremely efficient in terms of teacher time as, in so far as accommodation allows, the session can be delivered to large numbers of students at the same time. It is also a very useful way of introducing new topics, which may act as a motivator for the students. Further, the knowledge you provide can be totally up-to-date.

Finally, the lecture provides a useful framework on which to base other sessions. For example, the students may all be given the same information in a lecture, and may then break up into smaller groups to discuss it.

Some of the criticisms levelled at the lecture method are derogatory at best and are certainly not new. Auden (cited in Curzon 1997, p. 191), states that 'the lecturer is a person who talks in someone else's sleep'.

This might at first glance be a bit off-putting to the new lecturer, but should instil in us the need to make the subject we are going to teach of interest. Some other criticisms of the lecture method are that:

- The students are mainly passive (although the students may see this as a plus!).
- Lectures may not appeal to the student's individual learning style.
- The opportunity to explore the issues raised is limited.

Finally, it is difficult for the teacher to ascertain whether he or she has been understood.

Handouts

These are a very useful tool that provide students with a record of what you have taught during the lecture. They have the added advantage of enabling students to concentrate on what you are saying, rather than taking notes. Whether or not you use them, however, will depend on the time you have in which to prepare them and the facilities you have available to produce them. There are two basic types: the handout on which you provide all the key points of your lecture, and the gapped handout, which gives students the main headings and space between each one to enable them to complete it during the lecture.

There are five key areas that you should include in a handout:

1. The topic being taught

2. The aim and objectives (or learning outcomes) of the session

3. A statement of the main thrust of the presentation

4. A summary of the key points

5. An up-to-date list of further reading that students can access if they require more information.

If you were to present a lecture on the effects of smoking on health, a gapped handout would look something like Figure 2.1. The student then completes the handout from the information given during the lecture.

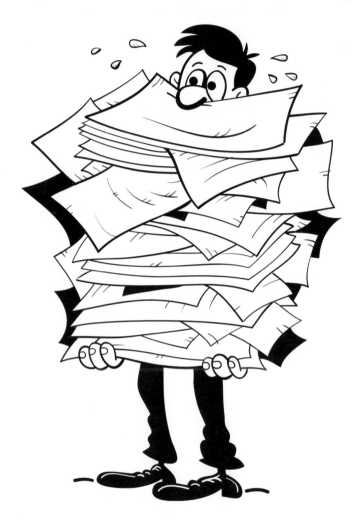

Delivering a lecture

There are seven basic steps that are useful to follow before delivering a lecture:

1. Planning what it is you are going to teach
2. Collecting and undertaking essential reading (what do you need to know in order to teach it effectively?)
3. Writing a detailed outline
4. Rehearsing
5. Selecting examples to illustrate your teaching

FIGURE 2.1	A gapped handout.

The effects of smoking on health

Learning objectives

At the end of the session students should be able to:

- Discuss the ways in which smoking affects health
- Describe two of the major health promotion models used to educate people regarding the dangers of smoking.

Questions

1   What are the effects of smoking on health in the following domains?
    Physical

    Social

    Psychological

    Economic

2   What are the major models used in health promotion?
    a

    b

Further reading

Provide a list of relevant material that the students will find useful.

6. Knowing and understanding the content

7. Selecting appropriate visual aids.

Varying your teaching methods will appeal to students' different learning styles, and even within the lecture you should try to introduce some change of activity – for example the use of audiovisual aids or gapped handouts – and allow time for questions during and after the session.

The next step is writing a detailed outline. There is a fine balance to be drawn here. First, it is tempting to write down all that you know on a particular subject, and then to read it to the group. This should be avoided at all costs, as it does not allow for student interaction and potentially makes the teaching session both short and boring. Furthermore, it gives the impression that the teacher wants to control the learners, rather than learning alongside them.

The preparation of teaching notes will help you to start planning your teaching session. You will find that the preparation is initially extremely time-consuming, but becomes much quicker with practice. Your teaching plan can also be updated, so it can be used again. As a result, your portfolio of prepared material is gradually built up, but don't forget to review your evidence-base constantly!

Your notes are also a very useful prompt when teaching, to keep you on course:

- Keep your notes reasonably short, but always include the outcomes or objectives for the session and explain their relevance.

- Highlight important points on your plan by using a highlighter pen or red ink. This will ensure you do not omit any information crucial to your teaching. ·

- Fasten your papers together securely, or ensure that they are adequately numbered (if you are extremely nervous and drop them, you will need to be able to reorder them quickly).

- Make sure that your plan follows a logical sequence, with a clear introduction, middle and end.

Use the introduction to outline what you intend to do and its relevance, the middle section to provide the new information and the summary to 'pull together' the main points. As the old adage runs: 'tell 'em what you're going to tell 'em; tell 'em; and then tell 'em what you've told 'em' (see Activity 2.2).

Now you are ready to rehearse your session. There are unfortunately no shortcuts to this, as timing is crucial if teaching is to be effective. Many of us have experienced the teaching session that has run way over time, leaving the students tense, irritable and totally switched off. The answer to this potential problem lies in rehearsal, possibly in front of a friend. The confidence that you can gain from doing this is tremendous. First, it enables you to become much more conversant with your subject matter, and second, it ensures that you will not run out of material in the first 5 minutes.

To illustrate the points you are making, you need to choose some practical examples from your own area of work. For example, if a community nurse is teaching about the safe storage of drugs in the client's home, it becomes much more meaningful to students if this can be applied to their own experiences, and so helps to bring the teaching to life.

When planning your presentation, it is always worth asking yourself what relevant examples you can use to link theory with practice, but beware of relying too heavily on stories from your own practice unless they are totally pertinent to what you are teaching.

An aspect of teaching you should never underestimate is knowing the content. This is probably the only place where no amount of strategic planning will help: you must have an understanding of your subject material and the major concepts involved. It is also useful (and will save you from embarrassment) if you have a reserve of knowledge over and above that which you are going to teach. By doing this, you will not be thrown off course by most questions the group may raise. On the other hand, there is no disgrace in a teacher not knowing the answer to a question, and to say so is far preferable to bluffing your way through. Thankfully, the days when a teacher was expected to know everything are long gone, but always find out the answer and get back to questioners.

One good practical tip for first-time teachers is to write out your key lecture points on cards fastened together with a strong elastic band. This will ensure that, if you are feeling particularly nervous and not quite in control of your hands, the notes will all fall to the floor together and will have stayed in the right order for you to pick them up and resume teaching where you left off!

Discussion and tutorial groups

These are best used when there are small groups of students. Between 12 and 15 is ideal, as larger numbers make it difficult to take individual contributions. This is a particularly useful method for enabling students to develop their skills in decision-making, but if it is to be successful as a teaching method, it is very important to ensure that all of the students are encouraged to participate.

The skills to ensure that individual students do not dominate and quiet students contribute grow with experience but it is always very useful to have a few questions 'up your sleeve' that you can address to any quiet members of the group to bring them into the discussion.

Tutorial groups

These are usually used as a back-up to information already being given by other methods. For example, a tutorial group may look at specific issues raised during a lecture, or may want to discuss the best way in which students can prepare themselves for an important examination. These groups are normally teacher-led, so the teacher needs a good understanding of what is to be discussed to enable the students to reach their conclusions.

Small group discussions are best suited to the following activities:

- Brainstorming
- Snowballing
- Buzz groups
- The presentation of projects or assignments
- Problem-solving.

Brainstorming

Brainstorming is a way of collecting ideas from all of the individuals in the group on how to deal with a particular problem. The students state their ideas on a particular issue, and these are then written down without comment or discussion.

However, if learning is to take place, the teacher must be clear about what he or she is trying to achieve.

When using this process the group needs to be clear on the type of idea they are being asked to produce. Examples might include:

- What are the advantages and disadvantages of using the lecture as a teaching method?
- What factors might encourage a patient to stop smoking?

The facilitator (teacher or student) asks the group for suggestions, and then writes them on the board as quickly as possible. No idea is excluded from the exercise, regardless of how irrelevant it may appear. By the same token, ideas should be recorded even if they have been previously suggested. No comment, judgement or discussion is entered into at this stage.

All suggestions are examined to ensure that there is a common understanding within the group of all the issues raised, and also to dispense with any ideas that the group feels inappropriate or does not wish to discuss.

Following this all remaining ideas are then discussed fully, and used to resolve the problem.

Brainstorming is very useful in enabling individual students to increase their confidence within the group. The speed at which the activity is undertaken does not allow students to consider how their idea will be received by the rest of the group, and also enables students to develop someone else's idea further.

More detail on the effectiveness of brainstorming can be found at www.businessballs.com/brainstorming.htm.

Snowballing

Snowballing involves the initial discussion of a subject in small groups; this then develops into a discussion in larger groups (just like a snowball that increases in size as it is rolled). This method has the added advantage that it can be used in larger groups of up to 32 students, as long as space is available.

The process starts with a clear statement of what is wanted from the group – for example, how can we help to ensure patients' and their visitors' personal safety while they are in hospital? Time is then given for each student to think about the issues individually. Their ideas are then combined with those of another student. Between them, they identify the similarities and differences in their ideas and what, if anything, they wish to reject. The pairs then snowball into groups of four, eight and finally 16, during which the issues are compared and discussed until a comprehensive answer is reached.

This is a particularly useful exercise if you are teaching a controversial subject (for example, the ethics of resources allocation), as one group may have to persuade another that their ideas are the 'right' ones.

Buzz groups

With buzz groups, students are divided into small groups of between two and six, and each is asked to discuss issues for a short period of time. An appointed reporter (often called a rapporteur) then feeds the information back to the group as a whole. To use the effects of smoking on health as an example, one group could be asked what the physical effects would be, one group the social effects, and so on.

Project presentation

Project presentation is a useful method to use if the subject you are teaching involves the discovery of information. For example, it may be about the function of a voluntary organisation that has been set up to support patients, or about drawing up a community profile. Students can work either singly or in groups. The information gained is presented and shared with the whole of the group, usually using audiovisual equipment.

The methods discussed so far are extremely useful in helping the quieter members of the group to grow in confidence, and in helping them to develop their interpersonal skills.

All of the above have two crucial elements that you, as the teacher, need to consider. First, the purpose of the session should be clear to the students, and second, students should feel comfortable and safe enough to contribute – for example, they should not feel that they are going to be made to look foolish in front of the group. There is undoubtedly an art in facilitating discussion groups that enables the teacher to support and get the best out of the students. This comes largely with experience.

Seminars

A seminar is particularly student-centred, as it involves the student presenting either a paper or an essay, following which a group discussion takes place. It is a useful method for exploring sociological issues – for example, the effects of social class on health, or ethical decision-making. While you as a teacher need a sound understanding of the subject material, it is useful to ask the student to formulate two or three questions from the presented paper which can then be discussed by the group.

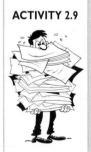

ACTIVITY 2.8

What aspects of teaching from your particular area of practice do you think would be best taught using the group discussion methods?

As identified above, group discussion is very useful for developing decision-making skills and changing attitudes. So, as an example, you could have selected a critical incident from your practice.

Role-play

Role-play is extremely useful in developing problem-solving skills and communication strategies, and in trying to change students' attitudes. It involves students playing the part of other people in a situation previously identified by the teacher. It is a method that, by its very nature, encourages active participation, scrutinises human behaviour and relationships and also helps students to understand the relationship between the ways in which they think and ways in which they feel. The fundamental belief of role-play is that because the students have gained a clearer understanding of themselves, it makes them more aware of the 'roles' adopted by the patients and clients in their care.

It is important to note, however, that the problems enacted may be artificial representations of real events, and the roles themselves may be so far exaggerated that they bear little resemblance to reality.

ACTIVITY 2.9

Think about your own learning experiences. Have you taken part in a role-play exercise? If so, did you find the experience enjoyable? If not, why do you think that was?

You may have found the experience stressful for many reasons. First, the fact that you were required to 'act' in front of the group may have been daunting. Second, you were required to 'make it up as you went along'; and third, you may have been asked to enact a role that you had difficulty relating to. I was once asked to take on the role of a Minister of War. As someone totally opposed to violence, I had some difficulty! It is therefore of vital importance when planning a role-play exercise that the students are comfortable with the process and that you, as a teacher, are sensitive to their needs. It may also be that the method does not meet the student's individual learning style, as identified in Chapter 1.

There are some key steps you may wish to take when planning your role-play:

- Identify clearly what you want the students to learn from the exercise.
- Provide the students with clear guidelines on the character each is to play, and his or her background.
- Keep the situation relatively simple, with no more than four players. If the situation is too complex, the teacher can miss some important issues when he or she comes to summarise.
- Give the role players time for preparation.
- Explain clearly to the audience the purpose of the session.
- Explore with the group the key issues raised in the role-play.

The following is an example of role-play and how it may assist learning. This scenario could be used to teach students the communication skills required when faced with behaviour that is difficult to deal with in practice.

A woman telephones the ward and demands to know why her admission has been cancelled. She is extremely angry.

The information given to student A would be as follows: You are a 55-year-old woman who has been on the waiting list for 4 months to have your gallbladder removed. You are frequently in a great deal of pain. You have just opened your morning's post to discover that the operation you were due to have tomorrow has been cancelled for the second time. This is despite the fact that you have undergone preoperative screening and you contacted the ward yesterday to confirm that it would go ahead. As a result you have reorganised your work commitments.

The information given to student B would be: You are in charge on a very busy surgical ward. The student nurse comes to tell you there is a woman on the phone who is very angry. The student says it seems that the woman was expecting to be admitted to the ward tomorrow for an operation, which has been cancelled, and wants to know what is going on.

A seemingly simple situation can provide rich opportunities for exploring different strategies for developing communication skills. However, when utilising role-play, it is important to provide the students with an opportunity to 'de-role' and also set aside ample time to discuss with the group what knowledge has been gained from the experience.

Learning from *critical incidents* is often used in the classroom in order to develop reflective practice. Although dated, Smith and Russell (1991, p. 289) provide an excellent example of the application of reflective practice to the teaching situation that involved the use of a journal which could still be of relevance to our practice today:

> Everyone was very busy. Sister told me to take [a patient's] wife a cup of tea and sit with her; the doctor would see her shortly. [The wife]

didn't know her husband had died. I felt sick. Mrs X asked me how her husband was. I kept saying I didn't know what had happened, but that the doctor would come soon and let her know. I was frightened she would know I was lying. I wished the doctor would hurry up.

This experience can then be used in the classroom to discuss issues relating to communication, the care of people who are dying and their relatives, and stress in nursing.

Self-directed/independent study

ACTIVITY 2.10

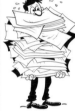

It is likely that in the past you have been taught using the self-directed/independent method. How useful did you find this in terms of your own learning? If you did not find that the method helped you to learn, why was this?

Based on your own experience, you will have your own views about self-directed or independent learning. There are a variety of views on its appropriateness as a teaching method.

There are two key elements to self-directed/independent learning that must be acknowledged if learning is to be effective:

1. Students take increasing responsibility for achieving the learning objectives or outcomes.
2. Students work at their own pace.

Fundamental to self-directed study is the need for adequate facilities – for example, the use of a comprehensive library and information technology. Most criticisms directed at this approach to learning centre on lack of resources. This is not always the case, however, and entire programmes of study are increasingly being developed in this way (see the section on online or e-learning later in this chapter). The level of student independence is largely determined by the course planners, who identify what is to be learned and how.

In view of this, there are degrees of self-directed/independent learning. In nursing education this tends to be a mixture of self- and teacher-directed, as it is recognised that courses leading to a nationally recognised qualification are rarely totally self-directed. This is particularly so in pre-registration courses in nursing, largely because of the criteria set down by the statutory body in order to maintain standards and patient safety.

ACTIVITY 2.11

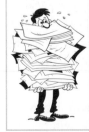

Think about your current role. Make a list of the activities that you think could be taught wholly self-directed, partly self-directed or wholly teacher-directed.

Self-directed learners become more experienced in working without close supervision. When they enter their jobs they are more confident of their own abilities and rely less on someone else to tell them what to do.

There are some tips that will help you to help your students to become more self-sufficient.

- Know your students well.
- Treat them with respect.
- Help them to identify their own learning needs.
- Acknowledge that you value their views.
- Try to ensure adequate resources.

Experiential learning

Experiential learning plays a key role in learning for many health professionals. In nursing, it is likely that much of your students' learning is experiential.

Experiential learning has a number of key elements:

- There is an emphasis on personal experience.
- It is an active process.
- Students are encouraged to reflect on, and therefore learn from, their own experiences.
- Experience is valued as a learning episode in itself.
- The facilitator/teacher adopts a supportive role in the learning process.

It is clear from the above that the prime place for this type of learning to occur is in practice.

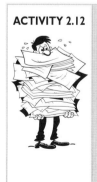

ACTIVITY 2.12

How can you, as a practitioner, facilitate experiential learning in students to whom you have been allocated? What factors do you think are important?

You have probably identified factors such as your own current knowledge and experience, the time available within your current role to support the student, and your knowledge of what the student already knows. It is important at this stage to note that, whereas curricula in nurse education combine theory and practice, the theory does not always come before the practice: students can learn equally well by gaining some of their experience in practice, and then learning the theory that underpins it. For example, it is possible for a student to be able to undertake a blood pressure recording safely without having a full understanding of the theory relating to hypotension and hypertension.

Online learning (e-learning) and teaching

If you enter the words 'online learning' into the search engine of your computer or laptop you will get hundreds of thousands of 'hits'. This is because the development in information technology has revolutionised the ways in which teachers are able to support student learning. The benefits of online learning as a credible way of improving and increasing knowledge cannot be underestimated and it now has a firm base in both pre- and post-registration curricula and also in supporting nurses in their continuing professional development. Online packages range from individual modules, e.g. anatomy and physiology, to complete programmes of study, such as diplomas.

ACTIVITY 2.13

Can you think of the benefits of online teaching materials for both the student and the teacher?

You may have listed some of the following:

- The virtual class size tends to be small (e.g. 12–20 per class) when compared with face-to-face teaching.
- Study can be undertaken at students' own speed (within reason, if it forms part of a wider module).
- Learning is available anywhere, everywhere at any time of the day or night.
- There are frequently opportunities to exchange ideas and network.
- Modules can be tailored to meet specific requirements.
- Results are often measurable and available on demand.

Online learning is invaluable but it is important to note that, in nursing, however effective these programmes or modules are, they need to be integrated and assessed as part of a whole (e.g. a pre-registration course), as currently in nursing it is not possible to undertake a pre-registration programme that is totally 'virtual'.

The use of audiovisual aids

There are many types of aid to help you in your teaching. First, it is useful to identify their value and purpose. Audiovisual aids and technology (in addition to online learning, outlined above) have several functions. They:

- Enhance the clarity of whatever you are trying to communicate
- Provide diversity in teaching methods
- Aid retention
- Give impact
- Simulate real-life situations
- Permit practice, and thus give confidence

- Use a range of senses
- Increase and sustain attention
- Provide realism
- Increase the meaningfulness of abstract concepts.

Most colleges of nursing have their own information technology or audiovisual department, able to offer specific advice. Although the following list is not exhaustive, it will provide you with an overview of what is available:

- Powerpoint
- Chalkboards (it is worth remembering that these are not easy to write on if you have never practised)
- Whiteboards (remember to use the correct markers that can be erased)
- Felt and magnetic boards
- Interactive DVDs/computerised programmes
- Charts and models
- Broadcasts
- Tape recordings
- Films
- Slide projectors.

When deciding whether to use an audiovisual aid, remember that it should not be used as an optional extra, or as the provider of the whole of the teaching that is to take place.

There are some fundamental questions to ask yourself before you make a final decision about the sort of audiovisual aid you want to use. Indeed, there are many other ways of helping students to retain information – for example, field trips, which are often an extremely enjoyable way of learning. It is crucial, however, that any visit is relevant to the learning and the theory that underpin it. For example, at an early point in their studies students gain tremendous benefit from discussing the concepts of primary healthcare in the university setting, and then following this up by a guided tour around a local health centre. The experience must be meaningful for the student if learning is to take place.

If your choice of teaching method is a lesson or lecture, Powerpoint (increasingly rarely backed up by transparencies in case the technology fails) is a very useful aid to the session. Its use can clarify key points for students, and assist them to make notes. Powerpoint has an added advantage for the nervous teacher, in that its use diverts students' attention from the teacher to the screen. There are some basic rules to follow in the preparation and use of Powerpoint, or indeed transparencies, if you are tempted to used the 'belt and braces' approach:

- Always use letters at least 1 cm high.
- Never use ordinary typewritten copy: on transparencies it is far too small for anyone sitting beyond the front row to see.
- If you are preparing material by hand, always use a strong base colour – for example, black and blue show up clearly. Red is often difficult to see. Note that often technology enables you to draw diagrams as you speak.
- Never put too many words on the Powerpoint. Six lines is probably the maximum for it not to look crowded.
- Resist the temptation to talk to the Powerpoint and ignore the students.
- Reveal information one point at a time. This will prevent students from writing everything down before they have had a chance to assimilate the information you are presenting.
- Try not to put every last word of your teaching material on Powerpoint or transparencies. Not only is it very boring for students, but it will also make your teaching stilted and unspontaneous.
- Give students time to write notes. Remember, a minute of silence is a long time for you, but not for the student who is trying to copy what you have written.
- Provide evidence for what you are saying.

Finally, always have a back-up plan of action. You may need this if the computer or projector light bulb fails. In order to save students from having to copy down what is on your Powerpoint or transparencies, you may want to prepare handouts of the content. If all goes well these can be given out at the end. However, in the event of faulty equipment, you can use the handouts as a framework for your session. Remember, if you do prepare handouts, tell the students at the start of the class that these are available to save them trying to copy everything down.

EVALUATING THE EFFECTIVENESS OF YOUR TEACHING

Evaluation of your teaching is key to the success of your student and to the processes of teaching, learning and assessment. It also makes a direct link with the development of aims and objectives identified earlier in this chapter, insomuch as you can evaluate how effective your teaching has been in delivering the objectives you specified.

Evaluation as a process

In order to evaluate learning and teaching effectively it is necessary to explore the following questions:

- Why do we need to evaluate?
- When is the best time to evaluate?
- Where is the most appropriate place to evaluate?
- What is it we need to evaluate?
- Who are we going to evaluate?
- How do we evaluate?

Why do we need to evaluate?

It is important to recognise that evaluation does not occur in a vacuum: it occurs throughout many different levels of the teaching and learning process.

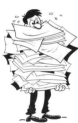

ACTIVITY 2.14 Take a few moments to reflect on why you think it is important for us to evaluate our teaching.

Your answers will probably include some of the following:

- To give us feedback on the quality of what we do
- To give us feedback on what the student has learned and/or achieved
- To assist in the shaping and reshaping of the curriculum
- To ensure that students are being taught at the right academic level (as identified in Chapter 1).

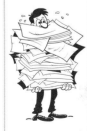

ACTIVITY 2.15 Now, from your personal experience of teaching and learning, as either a student or teacher, think about the different stages of evaluation you have come into contact with.

You may have identified some of the following:

- Professional course evaluation: Courses in nursing and midwifery have clear evaluation structures that enable teachers to ensure that they are meeting both the needs of the student and the outcomes set out for the course.
- Structures set up by government: For example, the publication of league tables by the government to identify which schools are meeting the standards they have set in higher education. (The Quality Assurance Agency for Higher Education (QAA) is charged with reviewing the quality of higher education. Its purpose is to get best value from the investment made by the public by setting up clear mechanisms for quality assurance.)

Consciously or subconsciously we all evaluate many aspects of our personal as well as our working lives. You might evaluate how effective your attempts at trying out a new recipe were, or how effective you think your son's new teacher is, or you may evaluate the delivery of client care or the process of teaching and learning.

The purpose of any evaluation is to improve upon outcomes, teaching processes or learning achievement, and ultimately to benefit patient/client care. We may also need to evaluate to ensure the cost-effectiveness of the delivery of learning.

In some circumstances, an evaluation process that identifies poor learning or poor client care may mean that drastic measures need to be taken, such as stopping an education programme or withdrawing students from a particular care environment. We may also need to submit a formal evaluation of teaching and learning in order to fulfil the requirements of specific educational programmes.

The process of evaluating teaching and learning should identify whether or not the teaching methods used were appropriate, whether the strategy to deliver the programme fitted the situation, whether the assessment methods used were the best choice for the topic or outcomes being assessed and, indeed, whether the learning outcomes had been developed correctly.

Evaluation may illustrate different aspects of what has been taught and what has been learned. It may demonstrate that the two do not match, and that failure to learn may result from the teaching process rather than the learning process. The process of evaluation provides everyone concerned with the information necessary to move forward.

How to evaluate your teaching

A number of methods can be used to evaluate learning and teaching, and, as you will find out, most can be used for both purposes. However, the aim of this section is to explore the evaluation of teaching. The following are forms of evaluation that can help you in this process.

Self-evaluation

Self-evaluation is a very useful way of helping you to identify personal progress. The Highland Council identifies some very clear purposes of a self evaluation system:

1. To encourage continuing self-evaluation and reflection and to promote an ongoing innovative approach to teaching

2. To encourage individual professional growth in areas of interest to the teacher

3. To improve teacher morale and motivation by treating teachers as professionals in charge of their own professional growth

4. To encourage teacher collegiality and discussion about practices amongst peers in a school

5. To support teachers as they experiment with instructional approaches that will move all students to higher levels of performance.

If, in your evaluation, you identify that some students have failed to learn, then something has gone wrong. It may be that the objectives, learning outcomes or components of the learning contract were unrealistic and did not fit the overall programme aims, or it may be that the methods used to deliver those outcomes were inappropriate to the learning style of the individual student.

Whatever has gone wrong, you will need to evaluate your methods and processes in order to identify the problem and correct it. If you do not evaluate yourself, there is a tendency to carry on as usual. The process of self-evaluation allows you to reflect and prepare yourself for future learning.

One useful way of self-evaluating your teaching is to undertake a SWOT and PEST analysis. SWOT stands for:

S   Strengths

W   Weaknesses

O   Opportunities

T   Threats.

Whereas PEST represents:

P   Political

E   Economic

S   Social

T   Technological.

Templates for both these activities are freely and readily available by entering the acronym into your search engine.

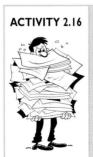

ACTIVITY 2.16

Undertake a SWOT analysis in relation to your role as a teacher.
   Your responses might be:

Strengths – confidence, enthusiasm, experience
Weaknesses – time, other competing commitments
Opportunities – working environment, teaching and/or assessor programme
Threats – work demands, other staff, other learners.

You are accountable to your learners to offer them the best opportunities to learn and progress.

One way to evaluate yourself is through a self-evaluation (or reflective) diary, and through the development of a personal professional portfolio (you will learn more about this in Chapter 4). As you are involved with updating and expanding your professional development as part of the NMC's post-registration education and practice (PREP) requirements, it is logical to use your development as a teacher to fulfil some of these requirements. A reflective diary, which not only details the processes you have gone through, but also shows how you have learned from these situations and improved your skills, will go some way towards meeting the NMC's requirements.

In *The PREP Handbook* (NMC 2006), it is suggested that you may wish to work through the following stages when planning your professional portfolio:

1. Review your competence. What are your strengths, areas that you need to develop, and areas for further personal development?

2. Set your learning objectives. What do you want to achieve?

3. Develop an action plan. What learning activities will help you to meet your needs?

4. Implement the action plan. Discuss your plan with your manager, link tutor or other relevant personnel.

5. Evaluate what happened. Once you have implemented the action plan, you can think about what happened and what you have learned.

6. Record your study time and learning outcomes. Accurately record all your learning activities.

All of these areas can be addressed in such a way as to encompass your teaching role, and the format should enable you to evaluate your techniques, your individual style and your development in relation to these skills, whilst at the same time meeting your PREP requirements.

Maintaining a personal professional portfolio enables you to keep a record of your professional development, whether in clinical practice or teaching. However, it is more than a record of achievement and should be based upon a regular process of reflection and, by implication, evaluation. The benefits of this process are numerous and include the development of analytical skills that you will be able to apply, not only to your own personal and professional growth, but also to the growth of others. Furthermore, such skills help you to assess your current standards of practice and to demonstrate experiential learning, all of which may allow you to obtain credit towards further qualifications.

In programmes that enable you to develop your teaching and assessing skills, this process of reflection can help you to evaluate yourself. Others will also assess you and evaluate your learning, as you will be observed by the tutors involved with course delivery, and their observation of your sessions will be documented.

Evaluative feedback

Evaluative feedback can be gained from a number of sources, via a wide range of methods. In many cases a variety of evaluation techniques are used in order to gain an overall view of the effectiveness of learning and teaching. Your evaluation processes will probably relate to a self-contained unit of learning, which will be specific to your clinical environment and the learners in it.

The outcome of evaluation should, therefore, aim to identify and demonstrate the appropriateness of:

- Teaching methods
- The structure adopted
- The implementation strategy
- Assessment methods
- The learning objectives.

The methods that can be used to ascertain these are:

- Checklists
- Interviews
- Questionnaires
- Results from learner assessment
- Feedback from other staff.

Use of any of these methods is an individual choice, but it is your responsibility to select the methods best suited to your needs. There is no single correct way to undertake evaluation. The methods selected may differ according to the aspect you wish to evaluate.

Checklists

Checklists can be used to start the self-evaluation process. A checklist should be seen as an aide-mémoire to the whole process of evaluation.

Most people are relatively familiar with a checklist approach. Think, for example, of when you go shopping and make a list; or when you prepare to undertake a clinical procedure and how you mentally (or physically) tick off the points as you go along. For example, when preparing to undertake an aseptic technique, your list might look like this:

- Trolley, appropriately prepared
- Dressing pack
- Cleansing solution
- Strapping

- Extra swabs/forceps
- Wound swab (just in case!).

However, when you prepare to undertake a teaching session your list may include:

- Room booked
- Learners aware of session, topic, time and place
- Teaching aids available
- Learning objectives prepared
- Audiovisual aids prepared
- Overall session prepared
- Self prepared!

This information can be gathered before you start a session and be fed into the whole evaluative process at the end. The next stage is to deliver the teaching session in question. During this session you will be able to ascertain whether or not it is going well. Intrinsic feedback can be gained from your activities; that is, you have an immediate idea of how you are performing, using such indicators as the learners' attention and the expression on their faces. This immediate feedback is important, as it might enable you to alter your presentation 'on the hoof', if possible, or to take this information into account when evaluating the whole session in order to make alterations for next time.

Interviews

A more formal method that you can use to evaluate your teaching is to question the group or individuals from the group. For this to be useful you need to ask specific and objective questions that can be answered by the individuals involved. It may be very difficult for learners to answer questions that need a personal response, especially about you, when they know that they will be working with you again and that you will be assessing their practice. It is best, therefore, if learners' evaluations concentrate on the teaching and learning process rather than on the teacher's competence. However, a structured interview may enable you to address some items in greater depth than questionnaires permit, and subsequent questions may develop because of responses to previous questions.

Interviews can be difficult to control at times, and it is all too easy to digress. In order to elicit the information required, it is advisable to prepare your questions in advance and set yourself a time limit for the interview. You will obviously need to record the outcomes of the interview. This could be done using an audiotape, with the student's permission, or by making notes during the activity. However, it is difficult to make notes when someone is talking: think back to the time you spent in a classroom, trying to make notes, and listen to and understand what was being said, all at the same time. Remember that you must be able to interpret the information later, when the student is not there to explain what he or she said or why, so make sure your notes are legible and comprehensive, and that you can understand them. Adequate preparation beforehand will greatly reduce any problems later.

Questionnaires

It may be more appropriate to devise a questionnaire to distribute to the group, especially where the content and process are the same and will be repeated with different individuals – by using this method you may be able to cover more aspects. Your questionnaire can be completed anonymously and be handed in for analysis and collation. The content must obviously apply to the topic and session concerned.

Ideally, you should use both open questions, which will need a written and therefore an individual response, and closed questions, which will require only a tick. Closed questions are easier to answer and easier to collate. By using questionnaires as an evaluation method you are undertaking research into your teaching, and by using both open and closed questions you are aiming to collect both qualitative and quantitative data.

The key to any questionnaire lies in its response rate (that is, the number of people who actually complete it as a percentage of those to whom it was given). A poor response rate will not give you a fair picture, so one way of aiming for a good response rate is to keep the questionnaire simple and answerable.

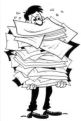

ACTIVITY 2.17

Consider any questionnaires that you might have completed in the past. What made some easy to complete? What made others difficult?
    Your responses to the first question might include:

- The length of the questionnaire
- The layout
- The language used;

and to the second question, your responses might be:

- Too long
- Too crowded
- Confusing/ambiguous language.

Ideally a questionnaire should take no longer than 4 or 5 minutes to complete, and telling respondents where to return the questionnaires is vital or you will not get them back.

You will need to decide when to distribute your questionnaire – either at the beginning or the end of your session. Whichever you choose, you need a speedy return of the completed forms, soon after the end of the session, in order to obtain an accurate response from your learners before failing memory or discussion with others can distort or alter the accuracy of their responses.

Once you have collected your completed questionnaires, you will need to collate and analyse the information obtained. You will probably be collecting both qualitative and quantitative data.

Once you have done this you may need to alter your session according to the results, repeat the session in its amended version, and then re-evaluate it. Remember that the process of evaluation and the development and redevelopment of your teaching should be an ongoing and cyclical process.

Evaluating the effectiveness of individual teaching sessions

So far we have looked at evaluation in relation to the wider issue of assessment and student feedback. This section will look specifically at the different evaluation methods you may wish to adopt before, during and after your teaching session.

When evaluating a teaching session, as mentioned earlier in this chapter the key questions for resolution are: what exactly are you going to evaluate and, probably more importantly, why? This is crucial, as it will ultimately determine the strategy you adopt.

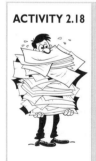

ACTIVITY 2.18

Make a list of the benefits you feel can be gained for both students and teachers by evaluating your teaching methods as opposed to what has been learned.

Under the 'student' heading you may have included aspects such as the 'feel-good factor'. The fact that the teacher is openly evaluating the effectiveness of his or her teaching often acts as a motivator, also providing the student with a clear picture of what he or she has learned.

For the teacher, evaluation provides an excellent framework for improving the session. For example, you may have incorporated role-play in your session and, following evaluation, now feel that a discussion group would have been more appropriate. Kiger (2004) believes that evaluation is an inevitable and essential part of the teaching–learning process.

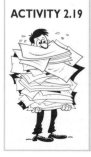

ACTIVITY 2.19

Kiger raises some very interesting points about evaluation. What do think she meant by the above statement? What does the statement mean to you? Why is it both inevitable and essential?

You may have included issues such as the students' opinion of the value of the teaching session, or whether the teacher felt that he or she had explained the subject in a way that was easily understood. Kiger terms this 'informal evaluation' and suggests that this takes place regardless of any strategic plan.

When broken down into component parts there are three aspects of the teaching session that can be effectively evaluated by the teacher: the plan, the process and the product.

Evaluating the teaching plan

This involves all of the preparation undertaken by the teacher prior to the teaching taking place. This may be a 'one-off' teaching session, in either the practice or the college environment, or a full course or module. It may appear almost contradictory to discuss evaluating a teaching session before it has begun, but there are many aspects of teaching that will greatly increase the likelihood of the content of the session or course being appropriate. To this end, there are some fundamental questions that you can ask once you have amassed your teaching material and clearly written your plan:

- Have you considered and included any instructions you have been given? For example, the session may be one of a sequence. If so, does your preparation follow on logically from the previous session and lead logically on to the next?

- Can you fulfil the objectives you have set for yourself with the content of the session?

- Will you be able to complete the session in the time you have been allocated?

- Is your teaching pitched at the right level for the group or student you are about to teach? For example, you would expect a third-year student to have a greater understanding of how to care for an unconscious patient than a first-year student.

- How confident are you with the teaching methods you will use? From Chapter 1, it is clear that using a variety of teaching methods both enhances the learning process and leads to a much more enjoyable learning experience.

- Are your objectives sufficiently clear to ensure that the student understands what is to be gained from the session?

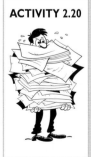

ACTIVITY 2.20   Take some time to think about how you could find out if you have fulfilled your objectives.

The most straightforward way is probably to ask the students. For example, you can pose a question directly relating to the objective and hope for an appropriate response. It is crucial to acknowledge, however, that it may only tell you that one student (or however many answer the question correctly) has an understanding, but it does not tell you about the whole class. Generally, it is valuable to use the first 5–10 minutes of any teaching session discussing with the students what they can expect to gain from it.

Evaluating the teaching process

A great deal of information can be gained by observation. This may be by the teacher delivering the session or by other teachers, when it is known as peer review.

Use of checklists/questionnaires in evaluation

A checklist is useful to enable you to identify aspects of your teaching that you could improve on, and it is particularly valuable when used at the same time as students' written evaluations.

There are many tools available to assist you in this, all of which identify five or six key areas for evaluation:

1. The teacher's presentation of the subject material: This involves the practical aspects of subject delivery, for example:

   - Could the teacher be heard?
   - Did the teaching follow a logical progression?
   - Was the teaching delivered in words that the students understood?
   - Were the visual aids used in the support of teaching clear and appropriate?

2. The teacher's approach to the students: This includes questions such as:

   - Was the teacher enthusiastic about the subject?
   - Was the teacher able to establish a rapport with the students?
   - Was the teacher able to recognise the need for student participation?
   - Did the teacher respond sensitively to the students?

3. Student understanding and participation:

   - Were the students encouraged effectively to become involved in the teaching session?
   - Was the learning related to the students' previous experience?
   - Was student interest maintained throughout the session?
   - Was the students' level of knowledge elicited at the start, in order to build on this?

4. Meeting objectives:

   - Were the objectives for the session discussed with the students?
   - Were the objectives appropriate?
   - Were the objectives specific and unambiguous?
   - Were the objectives shared with the students?

5. The teaching and learning environment:

   - Was the general environment conducive to learning, for example not too hot, too cold or too small?
   - Were surrounding noise levels acceptable?
   - Were the furnishings and teaching aids of an acceptable standard?

6. Feedback:

- Were students given immediate, appropriate and unambiguous feedback on the points they raised during the session?
- Were students advised on how they could improve their understanding and find out more information?

Using the above list as a framework you should be able to develop your own evaluation tool, which can then be adapted to meet any teaching situation, either in the classroom or the practice setting, and with individuals or groups.

Evaluating the teaching product

This type of evaluation tends to be more relevant to a course or module, as it involves more formal assessment and examination processes. For example, a high pass rate at examination is a reasonably good indicator that the product is satisfactory and that the criteria laid down for it are being met. Whatever the type of evaluation used, one aspect is fundamental to them all – that is, the need to act on the findings in order to improve the ways in which we teach.

CONCLUSION

This chapter has focused on the many factors that can affect the ways in which we teach and as a result influence the extent to which others learn. As has been identified, the fact that teaching and learning are so closely linked will also influence the way in which we evaluate our teaching in either the classroom or the practice setting. This chapter has also provided you with the basic information that you will need in order for you to teach effectively, either in your area of practice or in the classroom. It is not intended to provide you with an in-depth theoretical knowledge of the process of teaching and learning, but it should act as a reference point both to get you started and to provide you with the confidence to get over those last-minute nerves that, as teachers, we all experience from time to time.

REFERENCES

Concise Oxford Dictionary, 10th edn (1999) United States: Oxford University Press

Curzon L B (1997) Teaching in further education: an outline of principles and practice, 5th edn. London: Cassell

Hammer S, Collinson (2005) Achieving evidence based practice: a handbook for practitioners. Edinburgh: Churchill Livingstone

Highland Council. Available online at: http://www.highlandschoolsvirtualib.org.uk/ltt/lifelong/teacher_self.htm

Kiger A (2004) Teaching for health: the nurse as health educator, 3rd edn. Edinburgh: Churchill Livingstone/Elsevier

Nursing and Midwifery Council (2004) Standards of proficiency for pre-registration nursing education. London: NMC

Nursing and Midwifery Council (2006) The PREP handbook. London: NMC

Quinn F M, Hughes S J (2007) Quinn's principles and practice of nurse education, 5th edn. Cheltenham: Nelson Thornes

Smith A, Russell J (1991) Using critical learning: incidents in nurse education. Nurse Education Today 11: 284–291

3

How to use competencies in teaching

Dave Barton

CHAPTER CONTENTS

INTRODUCTION TO COMPETENCIES – DEFINITIONS AND TERMINOLOGY

> **LEARNING OBJECTIVES**
>
> The chapter seeks to enable particular outcomes for the novice teacher. By the end of this chapter you should be able to:
>
> ◆ Define and describe the term 'competency'
>
> ◆ Explain the principles of educational theory and practice in relation to the use of competencies
>
> ◆ Identify and describe competencies that are used in practice
>
> ◆ Describe and explain how competencies may be used to assist teaching, learning and mentors
>
> ◆ Describe and explain how and why competencies may be grouped together in frameworks.

The key intention of this chapter is to provide you, the teacher in the world of practice, with the knowledge and skill to understand and appreciate competencies, and how you may use them in your nursing practice. To that end, this chapter briefly explores key educational concepts and theoretical foundations, and relates these to the practical application of competencies in teaching. However, many of these foundation issues and themes may also be reviewed and explained elsewhere in this book and you will benefit from reading all of the chapters in developing your wider appreciation of the use of competencies.

In this chapter the aim and focus are always on competencies – how they are developed, their purpose in healthcare education and how can they be used by you, the practitioner. For consistency I will structure and describe competencies using the following simple standard headings (although note that there are many other alternative and similar structures elsewhere in the literature):

- Competency title
- Competency purpose and outcome
- Competency knowledge
- Competency skills
- Competency assessment

A competency on competencies!

It seems appropriate that this chapter, concerned as it is with competencies, be structured and subsequently defined in terms of a competency statement and competency outcome. Thus I provide you with a competency statement on competencies. In that way you may structure your learning on competencies, focus your knowledge and skills/ability acquisition as you progress through

BOX 3.1	A competency statement for using competencies	
	Competency title	Effective use of competencies in practice-based teaching
	Competency purpose and outcome	This competence is about the understanding and application of educational theories, their relation to competency statements and the subsequent use of competencies in the practice-based teaching context. It will enable you (the prospective teacher) to utilise competencies in enabling appropriate and effective teaching methods and effective curriculum/session design
		The assessment for this competency will be self-directed, and aimed at educational skill in the practice environment; it could form part of an informal or formal training or education programme developing educational expertise. The process should involve the delivery and evaluation of a predetermined skill acquisition teaching session(s)
		As eventual users of this competence you will need to ensure that your practice reflects up-to-date information and policies
	Competency knowledge	● Educational theory and practice ● Competencies – theory and practice ● Healthcare systems, skill mix and workforce planning ● Communication skills – and working with groups and individuals ● Specific specialist healthcare knowledge and skills
	Competency skills	You should be able to: ● Assess the student' learning role needs (e.g. skills acquisition – structured guidance) ● Assess the student's knowledge requirement and scope of practice ● Develop a personal portfolio and resource of learning material (e.g. develop teaching sessions, assessment strategies and tools) ● Develop a range of student learning activities and practice-based learning opportunities ● Implement, enact and evaluate a skills training session/programme ● Formatively and summatively measure and assess student performance ● Evaluate and respond to the student's learning experience and development ● Undertake critical peer and self-assessment
	Competency assessment	Defined teaching, student assessment tools, portfolio, observation, clinical simulation, formal evaluation, formal examination

the chapter, and finally be able to judge whether or not you have achieved a level of competence in competencies (I recommend that you study all the chapters in this book to attain this competence in full!).

Such competency statements, as illustrated in Box 3.1, are rather neat and attractive learning summaries for educators, employers and students. However, it is important that you understand that competencies may be presented in many diverse and differing ways, and may be very general, or very detailed. It is thus important not to take any presentation of any competency as absolute.

In response to that diversity, the following sections take a step-by-step approach through the concepts you will need to understand and use competencies in their varied forms. These sections will outline and signpost the theoretical foundations of education. More importantly, they will give working examples of how competencies are being used, and how they can be used in the practical teaching and clinical context.

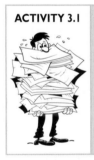

ACTIVITY 3.1

Think about a clinical practice skill that you are familiar with.
Write a list (no more than 10 points) of all the features and aspects of that skill.
If students were to read your skill list, would it help them understand that skill, and learn to use that skill?
Whether your answer is yes or no to the above – explain your answer!

What are competencies?

What is meant by the term 'competencies'? It is certainly a term that you will have heard widely used by healthcare staff and in healthcare organisations. For example, in the healthcare service of the 2000s, job descriptions are commonly accompanied by a list of 'desired' and 'required' competencies. Staff training days, and educational study courses, are today commonly accompanied by, and structured on, lists of competencies. Moreover, all who have worked in the UK healthcare or education sectors will be familiar with national occupational frameworks (exemplified by the Knowledge and Skills Framework–Department of Health 2004) and the National Qualifications Framework (Qualifications and Curriculum Authority 2008). These are competency frameworks used to structure and define organisations and their workforce profiles and needs. They are presented and characterised by daunting and weighty documents and are also commonly linked to extensive websites. All this brings seemingly endless instructions, rules, regulations, coding systems, and eventually bewildering lists of competencies.

Despite this apparent complexity, in simple terms competencies may be defined as the educational building blocks of occupational standards and descriptors. But, to the uninitiated or novice teacher who is trying for the first time to establish a simple programme of education for a specific need, competency frameworks can appear to be confusing and complicated. For example, competency frameworks rely on extensive educational vocabularies. Indeed, the terminologies associated with competencies can be very puzzling to the novice teacher, to the practitioner and to the student, as they are steeped in the theory and traditions of educational (and occupational) jargon. This is often further complicated by the inclusion of new and fashionable management jargon. There is often a (false) assumption made by experienced educationalists that everyone is familiar and fluent with these vocabularies, whereas in reality for many possible users of competencies it is a discipline full of words, terms and concepts that are at best only half understood! If that is the case the prospective user of competencies runs the risk of attempting to learn the educational theory, and apply those principles to practice, without basic fluency in the educational language and concepts.

Thus, you need a basic foundation in some of the most important terms and theories that you will most commonly encounter, and which underpin the use of competencies. But this chapter cannot give you a complete and comprehensive fluency in the theory and vocabulary of educational theory as it relates to competencies – for that you must augment your reading (see further reading list).

As a beginning, and at the most fundamental level, you must be sure that you understand the difference between 'competence', and 'competency' and 'competencies' and 'competency statements'. Are these words essentially the same, or are there significant differences between them? In addition, it is conceptually important to grasp that all four terms refer to a process, in that they may at once refer to educational beginnings (building blocks) as well as educational outcomes (Figure 3.1).

These terms may be defined in the following way:

- 'Competence' is a statement that describes the ability to do something adequately (regardless of the individual performing the skill).

- 'Competencies' are the plural of the above – a list or group of several statements that define an ability. Competencies are frequently grouped into common themes or domains which define a more complex activity or skill.

- 'Competency' is the observed behaviour that confirms an ability to do something adequately.

- A 'competence statement' is an educational term that refers to the written descriptor that outlines all features of the educational and learning process required to enable the competence.

FIGURE 3.1   *Learning and competencies – a process.*

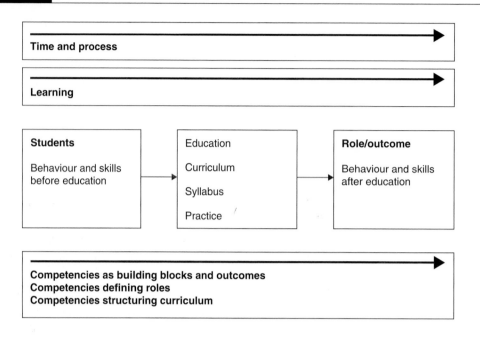

If we accept these definitions, then it follows that groups of competencies may be selectively drawn on, and that these groups of competencies may become increasingly complex, and may eventually define and structure entire occupational roles. Indeed, competency frameworks are actually used to define and structure large organisational workforces, planning skills and outcomes in complex organisations that deliver healthcare to large populations (Department of Health 2004).

However, before taking that step toward concepts of occupational and organisational role definition, consider first some of the principles and foundations of educational theory. For example, what tools are there available to us to measure a competence, and thus evaluate and judge eventual skill or role effectiveness? This type of questioning and thinking is crucial, and will lead you to further core educational concepts and vocabulary, e.g. curriculum, syllabus, assessment and examination (observation, essays, checklists, portfolios: Box 3.2). More questions will arise from this: where should we try to provide and measure a competence? In the practice setting, in the classroom, or in both? How often should we measure a competence? Just once, or twice, or perhaps many times? And do we expect competence to change, or should everyone be the same, or can we have levels (basic competence to expert competence)? What is clear is that, no matter how simple your initial concepts of education and competencies were, they will quickly and inexorably evolve to more and more complex concepts and questions!

BOX 3.2

The language of education

Education
The act or process of imparting or acquiring general knowledge, developing the powers of reasoning and judgement, and generally of preparing oneself or others intellectually for life

Teaching
The activity of educating or instructing or teaching; an activity that imparts knowledge or skill

Training
An activity leading to skilled behaviour

Learning
The cognitive process of acquiring skill or knowledge

Acquired behaviour

Aim
An anticipated outcome that is intended or that guides your planned actions

Objective
The goal intended to be attained

An intended learning outcome

Competence
The state or quality of being adequately or well-qualified or in possession of required skill, knowledge, qualification, or capacity

A competence is a statement that describes the ability to do something adequately (regardless of the individual performing the skill)

Competency
The observed behaviour that confirms an ability to do something adequately

Curriculum
An integrated course of academic and/or skills-based studies

Types of curriculum
Behavioural (outcome-driven competencies)

Experiential (learning from experience)

Apprenticeship (guided by an expert in practice to learn skill(s) or learning an occupation in practice)

Syllabus
An outline of the main points of a course of study, the subjects of a course of lectures, the contents of a curriculum

Assessment (see Chapter 5)
The act of judging or assessing a person or situation or event

Related terminology
Formative (developmental and/or diagnostic assessment – not usually included in the final grading). Summative–formal testing that produces marks and grades. Written assessment Portfolio assessment Observation assessment Oral assessment

Mentor (supervisor, clinical teacher, preceptor)
A wise and trusted counsellor or teacher

A person who supervises workers or the work done by others

An instructor

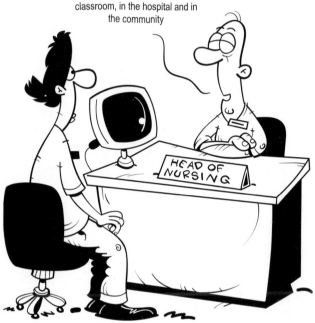

It's simple...all we need is a self-led curriculum that educates and trains the students within a multifaceted syllabus that is linked to a national competency framework that determines clear aims, objectives and performance criteria, meets national and local targets, is cost neutral, resource neutral, placement neutral and that mentors can formatively and summatively assess via the intranet and internet in the classroom, in the hospital and in the community

PRINCIPLES OF EDUCATION

Education is not a new concept or new practice. Literature on education goes back not just decades, and not even just centuries; indeed the origins of modern educational philosophy can be traced to ancient human civilisations (Curren 2000). Thus it is important to understand that there is a rich and diverse history of development in the theory and practice of education, and the understanding of education was not previously, and should not now be, confined to competencies alone. In reality, competencies as an educational concept and tool are newcomers to the world of education, or if you prefer they can be seen as a repackaging and refinement of older educational ideas. Many 'older-generation' teachers will recall hours of designing behavioural aims and objectives for their skills lessons, and will surely see these as little different from, or perhaps precursors to, more recent competency frameworks. It is important for the novice teacher to note that there are those who promote education frameworks (curricula) that focus on alternatives (experiential–humanistic) models of learning rather than solely on behavioural outcome models (competencies) (Ashworth 1992, Ashworth and Morrison 1991, Bechtel et al. 1999, Rischel et al. 2008).

Before we progress further, let us consider some of these basic and broad educational principles. These principles will allow you to use competencies wisely and effectively, acknowledging their advantages, but also their limitations. It follows that you should also understand that competencies are just one learning tool in the world of education or learning.

Education, it may be argued, is:

a guiding principle that enables the process by which societies, organisations and individuals develop and engage in valuable and meaningful social activity.

This statement will lend itself to extensive critique on the meaning of 'valuable' and 'meaningful' when this is contrasted with the complexity, diversity and consequent perspectives of human social order. However, the key points (words) that should engage you from this statement are those of 'principle' and 'process'. Education is a concept that rests on theoretical and practical principles and education is undoubtedly a process – it is a human activity that has to take a course and although there may be an outcome, education should not be defined by outcome alone.

In addition (and despite views to the contrary), education is not an experience confined to the few; in fact it is an experience that nearly all humans have encountered in one form or another. That may be by exposure as children to state education systems, instruction from our parents, guardians and social family units, influences from our friends and social lives, or from the role requirements of our work with professions or employers. Finally, there is the old theory that we are all products of the instructive education of general life experiences (the university of life). From this it may be reasonably deduced that we are all exposed continually in some way or other to the processes of education at all times, be that formal or not. Thus education, although a personal experience, is also a collective social and cultural experience (Figure 3.2).

In addition to this basic defining principle (education as a universal human experience) is the concept of education as a fundamental process of behavioural change. That process and outcome of behavioural change (an event that humans experience during and following the processes of education) is called learning. It can safely be agreed that learning is an experience we have all had! However, whilst education is usually described in positive terms, we must remember that learning may come in many guises:

- Learning as a positive experience (indeed, most educationalists and students would prefer that it were!), e.g. desirable learning – morality, social justice, fairness, altruism, human care (to name but a few)

The world of personal and individual learning.

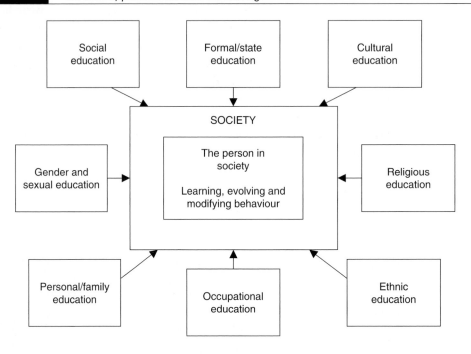

- Learning as a negative experience (it is quite possible for us to have negative learning experiences or to learn things that are not deemed useful in society's view), e.g. undesirable learning – avarice, deceit, aggression, malice (again, to name but a few).

Thus, although teaching and education may often be unsuccessful we must accept the central tenet of learning:

- It is contradictory to suggest that learning is ever unsuccessful. The student learns or does not learn – regardless of whether what has been learnt is considered desirable.

It is for this reason that human societies, in all their many forms, and in many different ways, take responsibility for controlling the process and principle and outcomes of education (curriculum), and making explicit what should be learnt (syllabus) in an attempt to achieve desirable outcomes in their citizens.

Let us examine in more detail what we mean by 'learning' – as any required competency will be inextricably tied to how learning enables the competency outcome. Learning is the experience and process of changing our behaviour as a result of new experiences, new skills, new knowledge, new roles. For example, children learn quickly that putting your hand into a fire is undesirable, indeed painful – they assimilate this new experience and new knowledge, and modify their future behaviour, by not trying it again. Thus they have changed, they learned, and they build on their social insights and behaviours. Equally, the healthcare practitioner may meet aggressive patients or clients; they interact, assimilate outcomes and learn to become progressively more competent in this skill. What is different here, between the child and adult, is that one is learning by chance and experimentation, whereas the other is being guided, and is receiving complex information and instruction from teachers and mentors. It is this structured educational experience with a predefined learning outcome that directs their learning (educates them) to an eventual occupational role (competence) that is generally viewed as desirable. It is the demands of this process (learning) of guidance (education) to desired outcomes that leads ultimately to the evolution of, and development of, occupational and professional competencies. Thus, in one sense, a competency is no more than this – a social need, skill or ability that is met by a desired outcome.

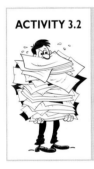

ACTIVITY 3.2

Think about the different types of learning that you have experienced.
In what way did they differ?
Write down your personal impressions and feelings of these different learning
  styles and experiences.
Ask your colleagues or students to do the same, and compare the answers they
  gave with yours.

THEORY AND PRACTICE OF EDUCATION

A key issue for any individual who is involved in education, either as a teacher or as a student, is the intimate relationship between the concepts of theory and practice. 'Theory' is the knowledge and concepts that are required to 'practise' a social, occupational, professional or academic activity. For example, chemists or physicists must acquire the knowledge of atoms, molecules and principles of mathematics if they are to practise their science. However, the acquisition of theory is no less important for those more social occupations that have a vocational (hands-on) aspect to their activity. In this case, the translation of theory into practice is a major concern for both educationalists and students. For example, it has long been known that the curriculum for healthcare occupations should contain varied aspects of the theory of human physiology and pathology, sociology, psychology and anthropology – these all often important theories and knowledge that varyingly underpin healthcare practice. It is the use and application of those theories in practice that are the concern. It has long been documented that a major educational failing in healthcare professions is the failure of theory being appropriately applied to practice, commonly referred to the 'theory–practice gap' (Upton 1999, Larsen et al. 2002). In simple terms, it is claimed that classroom teaching and theory bear no relation (and thus provide no benefit) to practice. Competencies address this required articulation of theory in practice; they tease out that link between the required knowledge-base, the enactment of practice and the assessment of ability.

A tried and tested practical solution to the theory–practice gap has been the use of traditional apprenticeship (vocational) approaches to education of healthcare professions. In this model students learn in practice – in a mentored capacity under the supervision of existing qualified experts. In practice learning presents in many forms – as long higher-education (university)-based programmes, or as further-education courses (National Vocational Qualifications or NVQs) or as employer-led training courses. The principles of apprenticeship curricula are commonly rooted in outcome models, and are increasingly dependent on competency frameworks. Apprenticeship curriculum models are evident in the medical and nursing professions, but are also commonly used in most of the allied health professions; they are also evident in the training of non-professional healthcare occupations. A key characteristic is the mix of theoretical input and practice exposures with defined outcomes (commonly competency-based). Such curricula are designed on core principles:

- The need for an over-riding philosophy behind the education process
- The syllabus of educational content
- The means of delivery of content (teaching)
- The need for theoretical teaching and educational experts
- The need for practice exposure and practice experts
- The assessment of outcome (competence, learning) in both theory and practice.

Curriculum (models) may vary, from humanistic experiential models to more structured behavioural models, and theorists will present many ways by which curricula may be constructed and used in practice (Kelly 2004, Pinar 2004). The range of this continuum will lead to discussion on the training and education divide – do we simply wish a student to perform as directed (be trained), or do we wish a more discerning thoughtful response (be educated) (Box 3.1)? The distinction may seem somewhat irrelevant, but it is one that will underpin the depth and breadth of any curriculum, and will be dependent on the outcome (competency) required. In simple terms it may be expedient to train a healthcare support worker, whereas it may be more appropriate to educate a nurse.

The demand of the health service user in recent years has increasingly placed the outcome of education at the heart of its needs. Whether those outcomes are high-level skills required of specialist medical or care staff, or whether they are more basic outcomes required of non-skilled health service staff, it is the desire of the service commissioners to have their workforce tailored and planned to meet specific service needs – to be 'fit for purpose'. Curricula that define outcomes in more general terms have been increasingly seen as inadequate in defining such outcomes, as lacking transferability between occupational groups, and as a consequence this has led to the rise of competencies as a defining mechanism of measuring educational requirements and more importantly as measuring skills and ability outcome.

WHY HAVE COMPETENCIES?

Healthcare is a complex process: it is a social service often based on extensive and complex organisational structures, served by multiple and varied occupations and professionals. The UK has an ideal example of such an organisation in its National Health Service (NHS). This giant of an organisation employs approximately 1.5 million staff with a budget of over £100 billion in 2008. It is a vast bureaucracy, with multiple component organisations, charged with a bewildering array of health-related and social care outcomes. Most importantly, in relation to competencies and role definitions, it is an organisation that is characterised by the division of labour. There is no one generic occupational group or profession that can meet the NHS labour demand. Consequently, it is a public service organisation dependent on the combined efforts of a diversity of non-skilled, skilled and specialist labour and each of these has a function – and all of them require education and/or training to achieve those functions.

Organisations, governments and employers are committed to the introduction of competencies as they increasingly link competencies to job profiles, and see them as a means of establishing occupational and quality indicators. Competencies enable this assessment, by supervisors, peers, subordinates and even patients. However the introduction of competencies into the healthcare workplace also places a burden of responsibility on employees and educators (key stakeholders) to see that they are fully and effectively implemented.

Competencies:

● Are (written) statements of human behaviour:

  – Psychomotor behaviour (technical and dexterity skills)
  – Cognitive behaviour (knowledge utilisation and interpretative skills)
  – Affective behaviour (human/social and interpersonal skills)

● Have four key components:

  1. Ability – the potential to perform specific tasks
  2. Knowledge – information acquired, developed or learned through formal or informal experience, study or investigation

3. Skill – the outcome of utilisation (enactment) of knowledge and ability
4. Proficiency – a measured competency based on an occupational role, the novice-to-expert continuum, and desired outcome.

● Have observable behavioural outcomes

● Have measurable outcomes

● Enable workforce, service, team and role design (and redesign)

● Enable employers and educators in strategic planning

● Enable programme/course/curriculum planning

● May be individualised or generalised.

In practice competencies have been used effectively in both the private and public healthcare sectors. They have proved to be important tools in

---

BOX 3.3	*A competency example*

Competency title (example): Assess older people's risk of falls

Competency purpose and outcome: including competency scope/performance criteria – intervention of individuals/patient and carers

This competence is about working directly with older people, and where appropriate with their carers, to assess their risk of falls. The assessment may be aimed at primary or secondary prevention of falls and may take place on an ad hoc basis or as part of a structured programme for identifying older people at risk of falls. The process should involve a holistic assessment of each individual and his or her specific needs. Users of this competence will need to ensure that practice reflects up-to-date information and policies

Competency knowledge

● Legal, professional and organisational requirements
● Consent and confidentiality
● Communication and relationships
● Working with individuals
● Health and well-being of older people
● Specialist healthcare knowledge and skills Record-keeping

Competency skills

● Assessing older people's risk of falls
● Assessing individuals' risk of osteoporosis

● Developing and agreeing individualised care plans with older people at risk of falls
● Implementing interventions with individuals at risk of osteoporosis
● Developing and agreeing individualised care plans with individuals at risk of osteoporosis
● Implementing interventions with older people at risk of falls
● Reviewing medication with older people

Competency assessment

A structured needs assessment using recognised assessment tools, which enables health professionals systematically to identify, record and promote the health and well-being of individuals enabling organisations to define their skill mix and structure their prospective workforce planning to enhance performance and outcome. Competencies can facilitate recruitment, job assessment, staff development and training, performance management, career planning and succession planning.

HOW TO USE COMPETENCIES

In the following section I summarise some practical examples of competencies (and competency frameworks) that are currently being used in education and in healthcare. It is of course very difficult in a text such as this to demonstrate a competency in action, as this is something that can only be fully realised in the practice environment.

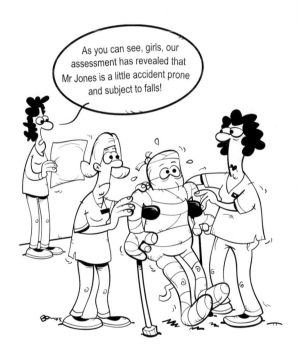

A competency example

To start, let us look at a competency drawn from the *Skills for Health* frameworks (Sector Skills Council for the UK Health Sect or 2008). This is an example of how a skill may be carefully detailed and described, and how each part of the learning may be outlined:

For the purposes of this chapter, this example (Box 3.3) has been refined and slimmed down. This is an important point for you to understand – that competencies in their totality can be extremely lengthy and detailed. When you come to use competencies this will become increasingly apparent. Competencies at their inception (at the very top level of their description) may be characterised by simple statements (headings) of required ability.

- Competency title
- Competency purpose and outcome
- Competency knowledge
- Competency skills
- Competency assessment.

However, as the competency is explored and detail is teased out in depth, the eventual completed descriptor emerges as a lengthy and complex one that details all aspects of the knowledge, skill and assessment that would be needed to give foundation to the competency.

The competency shown in Box 3.3 concerns itself with older people, and their known risk of falling. It is drawn from a long list of similar and linked competencies. All of these competencies can be sorted into groups, ultimately forming a detailed descriptor for an individual's job description or occupational role.

This example illustrates that any skill/ability may be described in detail. Indeed, this may be a criticism of competency frameworks, that they may become long-winded exercises in description, rather than enactments of practice. The sensible application of a competency to practice lies with the practice teacher who will see the translation of the competency into a living skill.

Competencies are widely used in many settings and below are given examples of competencies currently found in practice. These examples are just snapshots from much broader and complex competency frameworks.

ACTIVITY 3.3

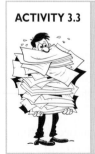

Identify a skill that you currently teach (or are planning to teach).
Write this skill out in a competency format.
Ask your colleagues or students to review and critique your competency.

Illustrations of competencies in use

Competencies used by professional regulators

Competencies have been widely used in professional regulatory processes in healthcare. For example, the Nursing and Midwifery Council (NMC) has included competencies in its Code (2008).

For example:

the people in your care must be able to trust you with their health and well-being. To justify that trust, you must:

- *Make the care of people your first concern, treating them as individuals and respecting their dignity*
- *Work with others to protect and promote the health and well-being of those in your care, their families and carers, and the wider community*
- *Provide a high standard of practice and care at all times*
- *Be open and honest, act with integrity and uphold the reputation of your profession.*

As a professional, you are personally accountable for actions and omissions in your practice and must always be able to justify your decisions.

You must always act lawfully, whether those laws relate to your professional practice or personal life

(extract from NMC 2008).

Competencies used in professional education

Competencies are widely used in all areas of adult education (universities and colleges). These organisations use competencies to structure their education programmes, enabling them to describe how curricula may be translated in to key measurable outcomes. Examples of these are competencies that are used as part of nurse education curricula at both pre- and post-qualification stages.

For example, the student should:

Demonstrate mastery in holistic assessment, diagnosis and management of a wide range of complex patient presentations
Demonstrate sound judgement in the execution of patient referrals
Develop and apply a theory-based conceptual framework to guide their clinical practice
Integrate the evidence-base to support and develop clinical practice

(extract from unpublished curriculum/module document, Swansea University 2005).

Competencies used by professional organisations

Professional organisations, such as the Royal College of Nursing (RCN), use competencies in a wide range of settings. A good example of this is the work that the RCN has undertaken in competencies for advanced clinical nursing practice.

For example, advanced nurse practitioners should:

Maintain current knowledge of their employing organisation and the financing of the healthcare system as it affects delivery of care.

They should participate in organisational decision-making, interpreting variations in. outcomes, and using data from information systems to improve practice.

Manage organisational functions and resources within the scope of responsibilities as defined in a job description

(extract from RCN 2007).

Competencies used by government

Government organisations use competencies in structuring, regulating and planning service needs. The most notable of these presently in the UK is the Sector Skills Council (SSC) for the UK health sector (*Skills for Health*). The remit of *Skills for Health* is to develop competency frameworks for the healthcare service to enable flexible workforce planning (Sector Skills Council for the UK Health Sector 2008).

For example, the practitioner should have:

A working understanding of how to read prescriptions/medication administration charts to identify:

The medication required.

The dose required.

The route for administration.

The time and frequency for administration.

A working understanding of how to prepare the medication for administration using a non-touch technique.

A working understanding of how you would check that the individual had taken their medication.

A working understanding of how you dispose of different medications

(extract from Sector Skills Council for the UK Health Sector 2008).

Competencies used by the NHS

The NHS Careers Framework (the NHS Knowledge and Skills Framework: NHS KSF (Department of Health 2004)) is a complex competency framework that sets out the various knowledge and skills which different staff require in order to function effectively. It is an embracing and transparent competency framework most commonly associated with the NHS career initiative known as Agenda for Change.

For example, the employee:

Communicates with a limited range of people on day-to-day matters in a form that is appropriate to them and the situation.
Reduces barriers to effective communication.
Presents a positive image of her/himself and the service.
Accurately reports and/or records work activities according to organisational procedures.
Communicates information only to those people who have the right and need to know it consistent with legislation, policies and procedures
(extract from Department of Health 2004).

Competencies used in primary, secondary and further education

These competencies include Credit and Qualifications Frameworks – National Qualifications Framework (NQF) in England, Northern Ireland and Wales; Scottish Credit and Qualifications Framework (SCQF); and Credit and Qualifications Framework for Wales (CQFW).

The NQF sorts national qualifications into three categories and nine levels. These include GCSEs, A levels and NVQs. The NQF seeks to set a national standard of educational access that will enhance motivation and enable lifelong learning.

For example, pupils should be able to:

Identify, select and use a range of historical sources, including textual, visual and oral sources, artefacts and the historic environment.
Evaluate the sources used in order to reach reasoned conclusions.
Present and organise accounts and explanations about the past that are coherent, structured and substantiated, using chronological conventions and historical vocabulary.
Communicate their knowledge and understanding of history in a variety of ways, using chronological conventions and historical vocabulary
(extract from National Curriculum 2008).

USING COMPETENCIES TO TEACH, MENTOR AND LEARN

One of the main points of this chapter is to explain how the teacher, the mentor and the student may use competencies in their teaching and learning activity. So far we have explored the principles and foundations which are essential for the user of competencies. I hope that it has become evident that competencies are tools that will guide what is taught, detail and describe the content of what is taught, and make transparent how assessment will be undertaken and performance measured. If we use the headings at the beginning of the chapter this will become clear.

Competency title

Teachers

A competency title is crucial; it defines the entire purpose and direction of the competency. Teachers can select, design and define the broad baseline intention of the skill they intend to teach the student. The titles of competencies are also important when groups of competencies are drawn together to form wider themes and frameworks.

Clinical mentors

The competency title makes clear to the clinical mentor what the student is expected to learn in practice.

Students

For the student the competency title is crucial in defining purpose and direction, but also in enabling the students' understanding of what they will gain from learning this competency.

An example of a competency title would be:

Skills for Health CHS23: Carry out intravenous infusion.

Competency purpose and outcome

Teachers

The teacher can use competencies to give a detailed description of what is to be taught to the student and other mentors. That description may be multilevel, ranging from broad aims and objectives to a detailed breakdown of behavioural outcomes.

Clinical mentors

This purpose and outcome guide mentors in their clinical instruction, allowing them to give direction and guide the level and scope of their teaching.

Students

This enables students to understand, rationalise and track their develop-ment in achieving the outcome of their learning. The student can draw on this to structure their learning opportunities in practice.

An example of a competency purpose would be:

> Skills for Health CHS23: Carry out intravenous infusion. This competence covers setting up equipment and attaching prescribed intravenous fluids to existing intravenous cannulae.
>
> This procedure may be performed with adults or children and will usually take place in hospital with individuals receiving healthcare. It may also take place in a therapeutic, research or emergency situation.

Competency skills

Teachers

The skill for the competency may be described in multilevel detail, review-ing all the contexts, facets, aspects and features that will need to be learnt for the competency to be achieved.

Clinical mentors

This gives mentors a clear guide as to the skill and ability the student is achieving, and on the contextual scope of that learning process.

Students

A clear statement of skill requirement will enable students to tailor their learning and assessment. Many students will be required to record with a clinical mentor their skill development in a variety of assessment strategies. The clear skill statement will enable them to achieve this.

Competency knowledge

Teachers

The teacher can detail all the areas of knowledge that will be required for the skill to be safely and appropriately undertaken. This detail should be evidence-based, be extensive and draw on multiple sources of research knowledge and theory.

Clinical mentors

It is important that the clinical mentor understands what theoretical preparation is expected of his or her student in order to gauge the use and application of this evidence-base to appropriate clinical skill development.

Students

Students can use the competency knowledge guidance to direct their study
in acquiring the correct level and appropriate evidence-based knowledge
for application and support of their skill acquisition.

Competency assessment

Teachers

The teacher can prescribe in advance to the student and mentors the assessment methods, theoretical and practical, that will be used, and his or her
expectation for the competency to be deemed to have been achieved. Tools
of assessment are detailed further in Chapter 5.

Clinical mentors

Assessment is a key issue for clinical mentors. They are usually the primary
focus in preparing students for assessment in the practice area and this area
of the competency will significantly structure that preparation.

Students

Most students are preoccupied with assessment – perhaps understandably,
as this is the measure by which they will be deemed to be competent, or
not. The clarity of assessment strategy afforded by the competency will
allow students to channel their skill development to achieve a successful
outcome.

The above has illustrated how teachers, students and clinical mentors
can utilise and benefit from just one competency. However, it is generally
unusual for a singular competency to be taught, as the student is more
often than not seeking to develop a wider occupational portfolio of skills
to meet the needs of a particular job description or professional role.

The final section of this chapter looks briefly at the competency frameworks that are now used to define, direct and measure these more complex
groupings.

WHAT IS A COMPETENCY FRAMEWORK/MODEL/SUITE?

As noted earlier, competencies are plagued by jargon and the reader may have encountered many different terms for collections or groups of competencies – frameworks, models and suites are just some titles currently in vogue. I have generally referred to these competency groups as frameworks. A competency framework is (in one sense) no more than a collection of competencies, often organised into categories or clusters. A competency framework would be designed and expected to be pertinent to an organisation, or to an occupational group within an organisation. We have already discussed how individual competencies define and support key skills, abilities and behaviours. However, competency frameworks are more complex, in that they may be general and apply to all employees, or alternatively they may only apply to specific occupations or roles.

For the employer, competency frameworks are a means of describing and defining the complex division of labour demanded in large skills-based organisations. They enable workforce planning, strategic direction, employee grading, staff development and quality control. However, for the educationalist, the teachers, mentors and students, competency frameworks take on a different guise. They enable learning and they direct and support teaching and assessment. For the teacher competencies are a key tool in modern curriculum design.

In addition, as competency frameworks have attracted so much government support, they are now freely available public domain resources that novice teachers may draw on to construct and guide their teaching. The crucial element is for the teacher to understand where these frameworks have arisen from, what purpose and service they provide, and their limitations as well as benefits.

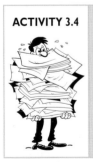

ACTIVITY 3.4

Select a competency framework that you are familiar with.
   Undertake a brief critique (review) of this framework
   List its potential advantages and disadvantages.
   Identify five ways in which this competency framework could improve your teaching practice.

CONCLUSION

This chapter has taken a tour of competencies: their theoretical foundations, definitions, purpose, advantages and disadvantages – specifically for the novice teacher who works in the practice setting.

Competencies are building blocks of teaching design and learning outcomes. They are ability statements that detail all that is required for the student and teacher to ensure that it is achieved. In the modern healthcare world they are now increasingly used to structure role definitions for individuals and whole occupational groups. Their value is that they define outcome, and as such can be used as tools of measurement in a working environment that is driven by the need to assure quality. Their disadvantages are that they should not be seen as the only mechanism by which learning may be achieved.

Within the limitations of a book such as this, it must be hoped that you now have the necessary insights and tools with which to begin your use of competency statements. However, in the complex world of education it need hardly be stated that wider reading will complement your proficiency in using competencies, and that competency use will be refined with practice.

REFERENCES

Ashworth P (1992) Being competent and having 'competencies'. Journal of Further and Higher Education 16: 8–17

Ashworth P, Morrison P (1991) Problems of competence-based nurse education. Nurse Education Today 11: 256–260

Bechtel G A, Davidhizar R, Bradshaw M J (1999) Problem-based learning in a competency-based world. Nurse Education Today 19: 182–187

Curren R (2000) Aristotle on the necessity of public education. Lanham, MD: Rowman & Littlefield

Department of Health (2004) The NHS knowledge and skills framework (NHS KSF) and the development review process. London: HMSO

Kelly A V (2004) The curriculum: theory and practice. London: Sage Publications

Larsen K, Adamsen L, Bjerregaard L et al. (2002) There is no gap 'per se' between theory and practice: research knowledge and clinical knowledge are developed in different contexts and follow their own logic. Nursing Outlook 50: 204–212

National Curriculum Online (History Key Stage Three) (2008) Available online at: http://www.nc.uk.ne/webdav/ harmonise?Page/@id=6016. Accessed on 11 March 2008

Nursing and Midwifery Council (2008) The code – standards of conduct, performance and ethics for nurses and midwives. London: NMC

Pinar W (2004) What is curriculum theory? New Jersey: Lawrence Erlbaum

Qualifications and Curriculum Authority (NCA) (2008) The national qualifications framework website. Available online at: http://www.qca.org.uk/qca_5967.aspx. Accessed on 11 March 2008

Rischel V, Larsen K, Jackson K (2008) Embodied dispositions or experience? Identifying new patterns of professional competence. Journal of Advanced Nursing 61: 512–521

Royal College of Nursing (2007) Guide to advanced practice. Available online at: http://www.rcn.org.uk/__data/assets/pdf_ file/0003/146478/003207.pdf. Accessed on 11 March 2008

Sector Skills Council for the UK Health Sector (2008) Skills for health. Available online at: http://www.skillsforhealth.org.uk/. Accessed on 11 March 2008

Upton D J (1999) How can we achieve evidence-based practice if we have a theory–practice gap in nursing today? Journal of Advanced Nursing 29: 549–555

FURTHER READING

Davis R, Turner E, Hicks D et al. (2007) Developing an integrated career and competency framework for diabetes nursing. Journal of Clinical Nursing 17: 168–174

This paper describes the development of a competency framework that relates to the demands of a specific pathology and client group (diabetes). As such it describes how the competency framework is designed for numerous levels of professional performance – from support worker to advanced practitioner.

Dolan G (2003) Assessing student nurse clinical competency: will we ever get it right? Journal of Clinical Nursing 12: 132–141

An interesting report on the implementation of a competency framework in a nurse education curriculum. The research reveals the need for ongoing revision and development to ensure rigour and consistency.

Irvine F (2005) Exploring district nursing competencies in health promotion: the use of the Delphi technique. Journal of Clinical Nursing 14: 965–975

This paper offers an insight to the introduction of a competency framework for a specific healthcare role (district nurses). A key finding is the demand for a framework that ranges across diverse performance outcomes, and also for the need for professional consensus of such a framework if it is to be effective.

Kleinman C S (2003) Leadership roles, competencies, and education: how prepared are our nurse managers? Journal of Nursing Administration 33: 451–455

This is an interesting paper that explores the issues and application of competencies to more senior healthcare management roles.

Maben J, Latter S, Macleod Clark J (2006) The theory–practice gap: impact of professional-bureaucratic work conflict on newly-qualified nurses. Journal of Advanced Nursing 55: 465–477

This is a useful paper that highlights the most current concerns regarding the translation of taught curriculum to practice. The paper critically reveals the current tensions and obstacles that exist between the educational ideal and the bureaucratic and organisational imperative.

Salonen A H, Kaunonen M, Meretoja R et al. (2007) Competence profiles of recently registered nurses working in intensive and emergency settings. Journal of Nursing Management 15: 792–800

This paper details how a competency scale may be used by clinical mentors in structured clinical development programmes. This is with particular reference to the management concerns of the healthcare organisation.

Watson R, Stimpson A, Topping A et al. (2002) Clinical competence assessment in nursing: a systematic review of the literature. Journal of Advanced Nursing 39: 421–431

This is a useful paper that acknowledges the topical use of competencies in healthcare education, whilst pointing to the demand for a more systemised research-based foundation in their application.

4 How to support learners

Sally Thomson

INTRODUCTION

Teaching is now an integral part of the registered nurse's role (Nursing and Midwifery Council 2008). Even though you may feel nervous about starting to teach, aim to give it your best shot, developing and refining your teaching skills all the time. We can all identify with the student nurse who may be apprehensive when starting work for the first time. (In our examples in this chapter we will assume the nurse is female.) She may be dreading certain sights and procedures. She may be terrified at having to cope with them. Her supernumerary status may leave her with unoccupied time and feelings of boredom or stress, especially if she does not know what to do or what is expected of her. To the student, you are unfamiliar – as is your work, your patients, your team and the ward routine. Think back to a placement that overawed you, and you can see how important you are in the student's life.

Pennington (2004) reflects: 'if we are unable to get the simple process of encouraging and supporting students right, then the future of nursing looks very grim indeed'.

LEARNING OBJECTIVES

After studying this chapter you should be able to:

◆ Work on your personal development, together with the development of your student. Aim to create a cycle of interchange between you as you work together

◆ Consider what you need to prepare for a student on placement

◆ Identify the significance of culture, socialisation and the respective roles of you and your student

◆ Explore some learning strategies to help both of you cope better with pressure

◆ Use the principles of mentoring to identify some strategies for communicating with your student, solving problems, giving her feedback, and finally, evaluating her placement.

The intention of this chapter is to foster a personal development approach for you and your students, as you both work together in your clinical practice. This approach will help you to evaluate the skills you already possess to support students on placement, and to identify those additional skills you need to develop. The purpose of this is to develop your talents and strengths, particularly when you help others to interpret and develop their own skills in clinical practice.

Each section of this chapter is interdependent upon the others. The order in which you read the sections does not matter, but occasionally you will find it impossible to avoid overlap with other sections. The chapter as a whole is intended to help you prepare satisfactorily for your role in helping students with their placement, providing a good experience for them during the placement, encouraging learning and working with your partners in the university team that prepares students to register as nurses.

The chapter is written as three sections: preparing yourself for the mentoring role, enacting this role and ending the mentoring relationship. It encourages you to reflect at each stage on your own role and that of your student – especially the ways in which you can learn together.

PREPARING YOURSELF FOR THE MENTORING ROLE

The NHS Modernisation Agency Leadership Centre (2004) identifies that the word 'mentor' comes from Greek mythology. Before setting out on his epic voyage, Ulysses entrusted his son to the care and direction of his old and trusted friend Mentor. However, young Telemachus' real mentor was the goddess Athena, who exhibited both warlike, challenging behaviours and the nurturing, supportive behaviours appropriate to the goddess of handicrafts and agriculture. These stretching and nurturing behaviours are at the heart of the mentoring relationship. If you want a quick and informative read on mentoring, this study guide is highly focused and helpful, as well as being easy to navigate your way around.

Modern mentoring has its origins in the concept of apprenticeship. In the days when the guilds ruled the commercial world, the road to business success began in an early apprenticeship to a master craftsman, trader or ship's captain (Modernisation Agency Leadership Centre 2004). This older, more experienced individual passed down his knowledge of how the task was done. This is very similar to how nursing and healthcare were taught and learned in the (apprenticeship) days before university-based education, and still underpins the principles of transmitting our craft to more inexperienced nurses today.

You should keep a personal portfolio of your work and its achievements. This will be a useful tool when you are marketing yourself to others, whether for job opportunities, courses, seeking funding for study or for your Knowledge and Skills Framework (KSF) review.

Your portfolio should acknowledge what you do well, and how you have grown in skills, knowledge and confidence. Confidence, which you may have worked hard to acquire, is what other people perceive in us – it is not necessarily how we feel about ourselves. McBrien's (2006) research found that staff nurses in particular often feel ill prepared for their teaching role. They may use avoidance tactics, rather than using this role to promote positive learning.

PORTFOLIOS AND PROFILES

A *portfolio* is a collection of evidence unique to you, which reflects your professional life, although some of it may be more private and personal. Typical portfolios may contain a statement of why nursing was chosen as a career, placement reports, old assignments, certificates, work contracts, assessment reports, significant pay slips, photographs, general life events such as marriage or starting a family, a record of any other critical events, and memorabilia such as letters of thanks, leaving cards, old badges and diaries. The portfolio must always include a curriculum vitae.

Including a leaving card in your portfolio is useful, because it can trigger reflections on why your career changed direction at that point.

Your portfolio should cover five or six themes that summarise your career development to date. These themes may include, for example, your teaching experience and ability or your clinical expertise. Your chosen themes will include information about yourself selected for a particular purpose, for instance to demonstrate that you meet the criteria of a role description.

A *profile*, however, is a more focused document. It is used for a particular purpose – for example, to demonstrate that you meet the criteria of a role description – and contains aspects of yourself and your career that you choose to make public. A profile is a tailor-made written source of information that summarises your experience and reflects your passions and interests. The profile summarises your career development, perhaps using the same five or six themes used in your portfolio, and reflects your main professional interests. It should grow and develop as your life and career progress. Your profile should portray yourself honestly – only you will know if you have done this. Reworking your profile can enhance your professional development, helping you to evaluate your experience and assess your career and mentoring role.

Begin writing your profile by looking at your current role description or that of the KSF attached to your post. Include your work in mentoring and supporting students, and draw up a list of experiences and activities relevant to this, including what you found useful when you were yourself a student. You may wish to consider how you develop your mentoring role, such as increasing confidence, achieving feedback on your role as a mentor and seeking any necessary support from colleagues. Even though this task can seem daunting when you start, it is well worthwhile because you will have a resource to use for job, course or university applications or, for example, putting yourself forward to speak at, or even to chair, conferences and so forth.

A personal development approach such as this will help you to achieve a clear focus on your learning, and to encourage others to do the same. It will assist your motivation, and help you set some personal goals and achieve them. It will help you develop your self-management skills, and provide a focus for your lifelong learning.

You will become less reliant on others to tell you how you are doing, and will be able to apply your learning and development to new contexts and situations. Your reflective approach will help you to develop the creative and analytical processes that underpin academic performance.

Secondly, a personal development approach will help you articulate your knowledge and skills, and (critically) see where you have used both in your work. It will help you to see what you are good at. It will assist you to make your career choices and future plans, by providing a useful tool for job applications or career development opportunities.

The first thing to do when considering how you support learners is to identify the behaviour that underpins this activity.

McBrien (2006) points out that engaging in clinical experience is a difficult adjustment for students. This stress can make concentration difficult, and may affect the student's ability to receive and process information. Consequently, a new and unfamiliar working environment or conditions can undermine the learning process for students since they may be tempted to abandon learning outcomes in favour of 'fitting in'. McBrien cites the statement 'I don't belong' as a familiar theme of student evaluations.

Friendly behaviour and an environment in which students feel safe to ask questions and to learn in their own ways will undoubtedly maximise the potential for clinical learning.

McBrien (2006) stresses the significance of creating an atmosphere where students feel they 'belong' and are accepted, so your attitude as mentor is critical to the socialisation of future nurses. Negative attitudes and lack of acceptance threaten the student's self-esteem and learning outcomes. To be blunt, they can make or break the student's perception of her clinical placement. Students felt staff nurses were pivotal for them in providing the link between theory and practice.

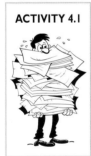

ACTIVITY 4.1

Consider what other people do that you interpret as support. How do those behaviours make you feel?

You should have identified a range of behaviours and emotions that rest upon communication, relationship skills and the feelings associated with 'fitting in'.

You may find it useful when reading this chapter to have the personal support of someone who can encourage and influence you, help you to reflect upon your practice, who is aware of and works with you on your skills development, and finally who will support you as your own mentor. Consider what skills you would look for in others to help you on your personal development journey. Now think who possesses those traits, or how you could find someone to support you as you support others. This person may be your clinical supervisor, senior nurse or your link tutor from the university. Or you may wish to explore with your manager how you could find such support, for example by networking.

By becoming a mentee at the same time as you mentor others, you will complete a learning circle of being mentored, reflecting on your own experience, and helping your student to evaluate her experience too.

ACTIVITY 4.2

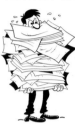

Complete the table below. This is designed to help you to apply your everyday skills to skills that support learners. Consider what you are good at and what you could improve upon. You may want to do this over a period of time, and return to it rather than doing it all at once now – try an approach based on themes.

Supporting skills and characteristics of a mentor	Examples of where or when you developed this skill/ understanding, or where you need to develop and how you might do this
Ability to form good relationships with others (positive communication skills) • Acting as a host • Acting as an advocate • Encouraging • Being resourceful • Confident • Approachable • Being a friend or 'buddy' • Making yourself available • Being helpful • Showing understanding • Welcoming	
Creating a safe environment for learning	
Accepting of others	
Helping others manage their feelings	
Being therapeutic in actions with patients	
Transmitting a passion for nursing	
Clinically competent and knowledgeable about area(s) of practice	
Motivated to give the best patient care	
Confident about teaching and assessment skills	
Providing a variety of learning opportunities	
A positive role model, practising from a strong value base	
Demonstrating mentoring and facilitation skills	

Now write an introductory paragraph for your curriculum vitae (CV), profile or portfolio that turns your list of skills into a paragraph. Look at your nursing posts over the last 3 years, and note your achievements in each area as you progressed through your career. Put these under your personal statement, noting the skills that you used to further your development.

You may want to use this in your first meeting with your mentor, by starting from the point of 'this is who I am and what I have done', before moving on to 'this is what I aspire to be'.

Now look at the Knowledge and Skills Framework and link these aspirations to your framework.

PREPARING FOR A STUDENT PLACEMENT

Material to collect before the student arrives

Firstly, identify the learning outcomes students are expected to demonstrate when on placement with you. Search for your university audit of the practice setting. How long ago was it written? Note the areas that were rated as successful, and any aspects that needed improvement. You may want to conduct a mini-review to see whether the ratings still apply, or whether there are significant variations between your findings and those found at the audit.

Additional material might include any formal or informal evaluations or feedback from students. Are there letters of thanks or criticism and what strengths or concerns do these express? What is your clinical learning environment like? For example, are there places where you could display educational material, such as unused notice boards? Is any of your material out-of-date? Has your practice area got a web page on the intranet? Are there existing learning resources, objectives or packs that can be used? Is there a teaching timetable, schedule or programme? Are there recent journal articles in your area of care that can be copied and shared with students?

At this stage, be sure that you have met the link person from the university and check if there are any link staff, placement coordinators or learning/practice facilitators able to support you in developing your skills and insights.

Price (2007) states that nurses consider their profession to be practice-based, and identifies clinical teaching and assessing as critical to the development of craft knowledge. He describes how skills in clinical practice integrate concepts, theory, critical thinking and research to develop the 'craft of nursing'. Nurses combine their practice observations, clinical experience, knowledge and skills to learn what nursing is.

'Craft' knowledge is used in practice, based both on experience and formal conceptual knowledge. So even if you might not be able to answer a student's particular question, you can still use and dispense your craft knowledge. This in turn requires feedback both on your performance and progress as a mentor and for the student of nursing. The promotion of craft knowledge depends on being able to link (and draw conclusions from) past experience, any current patient or clinical evidence and your theoretical knowledge.

The clinical culture

The culture of your working area will affect the student enormously. Cooper (2001), in her study of student learning, stresses the importance of the environment to student learning. She concludes that a positive relationship with qualified staff was the most important factor in the student experience, and that even the worst experiences were ameliorated by positive role models and sympathetic and supportive staff.

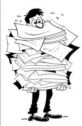

ACTIVITY 4.3

Consider the following themes as you work through this chapter:

- What learning outcomes does the student need to achieve? What does she need to learn? How can you add value to her stock of knowledge? What can you do to help her?
- What methods of learning in practice suit your student the best?
- How do the above match with your knowledge and expertise as a clinical nurse teacher? How can you best utilise the skills and knowledge you possess? How can you arrange for the student to learn about those areas that may not be your strength?
- Which aspects of your patient care are you proud of? How can you promote these?
- How do you use evidence-based practice? Is any of your practice deficient, for example not knowing what evidence supports the way you work? If this is the case, you should seek out the relevant National Institute for Health and Clinical Excellence (NICE) guidelines and clinical policies to refresh your memory.

This is all material to share and reflect upon with your mentor, and it will also help you prepare for your student's arrival for her placement and to feel ready for her.

Spouse (2001) reviewed research on how nursing students develop professional knowledge, stressing the importance of social support. She states that knowledge and understanding are both needed if students are to practise effectively. In her phenomenological study on learning to become a nurse, she describes how novice students initially rely on mentors, but with increasing confidence and self-direction they learn how to gain help from a variety of sources. She describes how students find it difficult to carry out procedures and relate to patients at the same time.

Students are concerned about how to manage what may be strong feelings and emotions, while at the same time adopting a professional approach to patients.

Significantly, how the student perceived herself as a nurse depended upon her acceptance by her colleagues.

Spouse (2001) identified seven categories of knowledge:

1. Relating to patients and relatives

2. Developing technical knowledge

3. Learning to bundle together activities of nursing

4. Developing craft knowledge

5. Functioning within a clinical team

6. Managing feelings and emotions (the student's as well as those of patients and relatives)

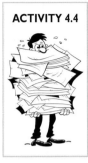

ACTIVITY 4.4

Link these seven categories of knowledge to the learning outcomes of the previous activity. By developing each part of your response, you will have a powerful matrix of learning from which to work.

7. Developing the essence of nursing that promotes therapeutic action (when the nursing intervention helps the patient).

In addition, Spouse (2001) found that students placed little value on routine work such as bathing the patient, as they tended to believe that they were competent in such work. Spouse describes how coaching and shared planning can help with teaching nurses the psychomotor skills involved in caring for groups of patients with different levels of dependence. She also concluded that students had fears of becoming 'hardened' in their attitude to clinical incidents, and found it difficult to reconcile the more detached approach of some staff to such incidents, tending to regard these staff as hard-hearted. So if your student is not going to get bored by routine work, ask her to find out something specific about the person she is caring for, that patient's clinical symptoms, how the individual is adapting to his or her illness, what the patient's job is, or perhaps how the individual lives his or her life. All this will help the student to see the patient 'in the round' – not just as a collection of symptoms.

If the student has trouble in planning a care programme for patients at different stages of illness, try to work out a timetable to give her a structured approach.

Spouse (2001) found that experienced practitioners use a body of knowledge built up over time. This is derived from practical everyday experience, often informed by theory. A successful clinical teacher will 'unlock' this knowledge when working collaboratively with her students.

You should reflect how you can structure the various areas of learning with your students, maximising the essence of Spouse's findings. As you work with your mentor, you may wish to look at how you can explore your own feelings to help students generate their coping strategies.

In 1980, Fretwell undertook a seminal piece of work exploring the ward learning environment. Despite the length of time and the many changes in nursing since this research, her central messages are still as applicable today. No chapter on supporting students would be complete without it. Her research demonstrated that students perceived the ward sister as the key teacher. In wards where the sister taught or showed a keen interest in teaching, other qualified staff members would do the same. In addition, placement students on such wards were very aware of this dedication to teaching. The ward sister would set the atmosphere and climate of the ward, thus influencing the climate of teaching and learning.

Some ward sisters were reluctant to take part in teaching and learning because they felt insecure, doubted their knowledge or were inhibited by their lack of teaching ability. In such cases, the ward sister might have a strong commitment to patients which took priority over that to students.

Students in Fretwell's (1980) study were the keenest to learn procedures and techniques focusing upon the technical aspects of care. Basic nursing activities were seen as work rather than learning and, despite the intervening years, things had not changed much, as seen from the findings of Spouse in 2001.

Fretwell's (1980) study described the attributes of the ward sister and her qualified colleagues in those wards where teaching was given high priority. These included:

- Showing an interest in the students when they start on the ward
- Ensuring good learner–staff relationships
- Being approachable, available, pleasant yet strict
- Promoting good staff and patient relationships and good quality of care
- Giving support and help to students
- Inviting questions and giving answers
- Helping and encouraging the students in their work
- Working as a team.

The features of successful ward teaching included:

- Discussing non-technical material, such as the patient's diagnosis and treatment needs
- All trained nurses teaching regularly
- 'Outsiders', including doctors and lecturers, also teaching regularly
- Senior students teaching
- Trained staff assessing students
- A programme of training and instruction
- Trained nurses teaching during the drug round and by example
- Students being given the opportunity to watch and perform new procedures
- Teaching and learning having a place in the routine

- Students being allowed on doctors' rounds
- Students being given opportunities to use textbooks and case notes
- Students being given responsibilities.

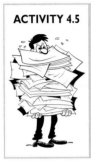

ACTIVITY 4.5

Now return to your notes in Activity 4.4 and add to them.

Devise a work-plan of things that you could develop as teaching opportunities. This may be a timetable or rota, or mapping opportunities for learning such as the ward round. Share the tasks out among your peers, set deadlines for completion and progress-chase.

Socialisation

Socialisation is the lifelong process that teaches us how different groups work, how individuals function within them and how to deal with new experiences. Part of your role as mentor is to socialise students into your working group and impress upon them its values and culture.

We can be socialised into ways of behaving without being aware of the process, since socialisation occurs whenever people interact with one another. Each person in an interaction influences the other.

Woodward (2003) says that role modelling takes place within groups. This is a powerful method of socialisation, and is the most common way that nurses learn. During this process of watching and copying others, students refine their own professional behaviour. The student uses role modelling to interpret her perception of the patient's world, and the part she plays in it.

Role modelling, which relies heavily on imitation, can be positive or negative. So, for example, observing negative behaviour means that students can adopt those traits if the role model has high status for the student. A student is not consciously aware that she has learned negative behaviour until a similar situation arises, when she may adopt the poor practice that was demonstrated on the previous occasion.

Work groups

Work groups are made up of individuals of all personality types, age ranges, ethnic backgrounds, cultural diversity, skills, intelligence and values. Work groups have to communicate with one another, in order to coordinate their activities as they work towards a shared goal.

Members of groups have different roles, status and power. They will conform to a greater or lesser extent to the group norms which form the code of conduct for that group.

Members of a group have, by definition, a sense of belonging to it. Think about the different professional and social groups that you belong to, and compare your motivation for being in each group, the different codes of conduct that exist within different groups, what happens if you behave differently to the norms of a particular group (i.e. exhibit deviant behaviour) and how other group members would then respond.

Norms are the established uniform behaviours of a group, ensuring that there is consistency and a certain predictability of action by different group members.

Norms link to group rules, which tend to be set (formally or informally) by group members with high status.

There is much further information about groups in books on social psychology and on the internet, and it is well worthwhile carrying out some research if you are interested in this topic.

People do not act only as individuals, since we are all influenced by the people we mix with in our work, social and domestic life. In everyday situations, we behave in ways that fit the particular context we are in; there are family, group, cultural, social or other expectations about the 'proper' way to behave. Meeting these expectations is essential if we are to be accepted by the group. Hence, groups will usually have sanctions that put pressure on individuals to behave in a way that conforms to the group's norms. Sanctions can vary from innuendo (which may be difficult to identify), mild or sterner rebukes from colleagues or even bullying or social isolation.

Sanctions can be formal (disciplinary procedures) or informal (peer-group pressure). Often, informal sanctions are the most difficult for a person to handle. Since it is human nature to want to be accepted by the group, the individual who is at risk of not conforming may find sanctions to be painful and may change her behaviour to ensure that she is accepted by the group. This may have a direct effect upon the standards of care to which a student nurse aspires, and will certainly affect her job satisfaction. For example, a student may be carrying out a procedure to the letter, whereas on the ward staff may cut corners to get the work done in time. The student may be aware of your frustration, not understanding what she is doing wrong and also may start to cut corners to ease the tension.

The culture of an organisation affects communication, social relations, individual actions and motivations, and also influences the rules, perspectives and ethical norms by which people work (Hecht et al. 2005). The consistent, permanent and long-standing members of a group tend to determine the group's norms and ways of working, which in turn affects the group members' working relationships.

We may all be able to recall experiences where the senior nurse in an area was a 'dragon' and how stressful and miserable that could make life; or how welcome it was to have a supportive person in charge of the team making the day meaningful and fun. Clearly, the working atmosphere will vary between clinical areas, teams and wards, and will also depend on which nurses are working on a shift. Members of a multiprofessional team visiting the ward may behave differently as they engage with the norms of different groups. In all cases, your role in providing student support is key to socialisation, since it is from you that the student learns how to nurse, what standards to adopt and how to relate to colleagues, patients and visitors. Poor nursing practice can desensitise students to basic human needs, and so your responsibility to the student is critical in ensuring that good nursing standards are achieved.

Hecht et al. (2005) also describe how the underlying values, beliefs and principles that underlie an organisation both exemplify and reinforce the basic principles of that culture with which the organisation's staff are expected to comply.

ACTIVITY 4.6

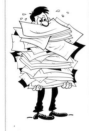

What values, beliefs and principles does your ward or team transmit about:

- Care?
- Nursing?
- Learning?

How would a student or visitor to your ward appreciate the above from interpreting your behaviour? Do you have a ward philosophy that clarifies and states this belief system?

Write down what you believe matters in these three areas. Use this as the basis of discussion with your mentor. Compare your priorities and beliefs with your mentor's, refining them after discussion, and including them in your portfolio.

You may wish to draft a position statement on the above lines to your team as a basis for discussion, and perhaps include any statement of values or objectives provided by the university. The aim should be to provide a succinct statement of your values in the three areas of care, nursing and learning, and to make this available to your students.

Consider how your values, beliefs and principles influence care, and how they may affect a student on placement. For example, you might include your values statement in an information pack for new students. You could also consider providing some background on what to expect in the first few days of the placement, using feedback from previous students ending their placement.

Your departing students might be asked to structure their comments by focusing on how you appear to others, your standards, the way you work, how you communicate with others and so on. You may wish to ask your mentor to do the same thing, and compare the statements.

The culture of the clinical team influences behaviour (what is acceptable and what is not). Unless students are aware of what behaviour is expected they will feel ill at ease and anxious. For instance, take a ward where the senior nurse always started the early-morning shift before it was scheduled, arriving on the ward at 7.00 A.M. whilst the night staff were still working on the handover. Other nurses on the ward complied with this unwritten norm almost without realising they were doing it. Newcomers to the ward, who were unaware of this, would arrive at the start of the shift at 7.45 A.M. They began to feel anxious about why they felt late for work, missing things such as bed-making and so on. They might incur informal sanctions from other nurses who felt that the newcomers were skiving and not complying with the ward norm.

Culture is complex: it includes membership of a family group, religious beliefs, social class, gender, ethnicity and age, as well as work groups.

Social behaviour is changed when people interact with each other. Each person in the interaction will influence the behaviour of the other, with pressure to achieve conformity and compliance.

Conformity

Conformity means that members of a group behave in a similar way to others, and the pressure to conform is a powerful influence on new members of a group. The power of the uniform and the prevailing attitudes of care in a clinical environment have a significant impact upon how a new group member behaves. Once new entrants to a care setting have assessed the prevailing values, they are able to develop a sense of belonging to their group. A new entrant to a group may be anxious until she can accurately identify the value system and accepted way of behaving. As mentor you have an obvious responsibility here to help ease the transition into your group.

Compliance

Compliance is a more complex process. It occurs when members of a group behave in the same way as other members of the group, but are uncomfortable doing so. Non-compliant individuals can feel scapegoated. For example, a senior nurse who is negative about the skills of a junior doctor may influence her staff to adopt similar unhelpful attitudes and behaviour towards that doctor. On the other hand, adopting a positive approach may carry others along on a wave of contagious goodwill.

The danger of compliance is that eventually a person may come to adopt the values that underpin the compliant behaviour, almost without thinking about it. Compliance with peer pressure leads to conformity. The needs to conform and comply are powerful tools when you are trying to bring about change and improve standards. In socialising your students into your group values, use briefings, debriefings, giving feedback on performance and offering alternative behaviours to undesirable conduct.

These are all examples of efforts made to achieve the desired conformity and compliance. The significance of mentoring and supervision is critical. Encouraging new students to keep reflective diaries and give feedback to you will highlight the issues arising during the students' induction.

Culture is crucial to the way we are socialised and socialise others into work. The prevailing culture can influence a person's self-esteem and generate positive or negative self-perception. To consider the influence of the culture you work in, the way it has developed, and how you contribute to it is to appreciate the importance of the social context upon an individual's behaviour.

The team culture will influence the daily lifestyle and behaviour of its members.

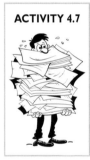

ACTIVITY 4.7

- Try writing down the unwritten rules that apply in your area, for example how coffee breaks are taken, how uniform is worn, how the doctors and other hospital colleagues are treated, visitors, the daily routine and the way care is delivered.
- How can you let students know these unwritten rules exist? If they don't appreciate these norms, they cannot make appropriate choices about their own behaviour.

Most of us find out that we have broken some unwritten rule, experiencing attempts by our peers to exert social control. To do this, other group members may use informal sanctions, comments, looks or exclusion tactics. Any of these can make the newcomer very unhappy if she does not know what unwritten rule is being broken. Therefore, it is essential that you think about what people need to know in order to survive in your culture and its associated codes of conduct.

Subgroups exist within team cultures. These can form and grow through a shared interest, research or outside work. They may form a social set or a group of deviants who exert pressure on others, and often impede progress or moves to change and develop work in your area. Comparing group behaviours makes it obvious that each subgroup has a different ethos, set of standards and purpose. An individual's behaviour and use of language within one group can be compared to the same person's behaviour and use of language when in another group. The various messages sent out can be conflicting. No wonder a newcomer can be confused as we switch between subgroups all the time.

Team members who have formed a social set can be easy to work with, since their good relationship skills will ensure that any issues can be resolved in an adult manner with goodwill and enthusiasm. In contrast, deviants are less easy to work with and may be harder to relate to. They can cause you and your nursing student to feel deskilled and apprehensive. Communication is critical in group processes, as well as an awareness of the impact that others have upon you. If you are aware of your place on a continuum from 'highly motivated' to 'totally put down', you may be better placed to assess how your student may feel and offer all necessary support.

There is much evidence to show that people behave according to the expectations of others. If people are treated as inferior, they will respond in a way that reinforces that perception. If people are valued, this results in healthy adult professional relationships that minimise tensions and underpin acceptable codes of behaviour.

Coon (1998) describes the importance of understanding other groups, since the insight gained can help to reduce tension and conflict. This is particularly true when you are trying to understand students who operate and study in an academic culture very different from the clinical environment. This should help you to understand potential role conflict and students' behaviour on the ward, allowing you to manage any conflict in a positive way before it gets worse and damages work relationships.

Consider a student shadowing you when you are particularly busy and working under pressure. The student needs to know if she can ask questions at the time, or must wait until later. The student needs to know what she can do to help you, as there is nothing worse for a student than to see the trained staff running around trying to get the work done while the student feels that she does not know what to do.

Roles

All members of society are given position or status by their culture. Sociologists differentiate between *ascribed* status, usually fixed at birth (e.g. gender and race) and *achieved* status, which means that the individual has gained control over his or her particular job and enjoys a certain position within his or her group.

Society expects those of a certain status to behave in a particular way. A set of norms (a role) is imposed on members with that status. For example, the role of the nurse is accompanied by a set of expectations about nursing behaviour. A role has been defined as 'a set of obligations and expectations' (Moore et al. 2005). Three assumptions exist about roles:

1. The *expected* role is the behaviour others expect that the role-holder should engage in.

2. The *perceived* role is the way the role-holder perceives that he or she should behave.

3. The *enacted* role is the actual behaviour that the role-holder adopts in his or her work.

When these three roles are in harmony there are very few problems, but when there is disparity between them members of a group will exert pressure to achieve conformity. The role we adopt in a group affects the way we relate to others, and the ways others communicate with us.

Explore your expectations of the student role with your students, covering the different behaviours required at the university and in clinical practice. It would also be instructive to compare your and their different perceptions of the role of the mentor.

Role conflict occurs when the pressure of one role overlaps with another, for example parenting, partnering and work. The role of leader or nurse may interfere with the role of mentor, and then strain occurs.

Dividing time between the student and patient is difficult when you are busy, and may cause you some role conflict as you try to give clinical care and also cope with the needs of an anxious student. Or you might be trying to sort out a problem with your manager when an emergency admission arrives, and you cannot then make a critical telephone call.

So at times of staff shortage, increasing volumes of work and the growing complexity of care, it is quite likely that role conflict and strain will also be evident.

ACTIVITY 4.8

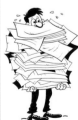

Write down the issues that cause you role conflict. Some of these might be your role outside work as a single person, carer, partner or parent. Some may be about the pressures you experience at work and the conflict this causes.

- Take these issues to your next mentoring session, and talk with your mentor about how to find personal compromises for yourself.
- Discuss with your students anything they feel makes it difficult to work in your clinical area, and encourage them to think how to ameliorate any difficulties.
- Compare your role with that of a student, looking for areas of conflict and compliance in core values.
- Work together to discuss the differences between being a patient, being a student and being a staff member in the practice setting. Identify your personal strengths and the student's. Encourage your student to set objectives around her relationship skills, and consider your own.

Northouse and Northouse (1998) identify four problems which disrupt communication between health professionals and between health professionals and patients:

1. Role uncertainty: there needs to be a level of agreement about what is expected of each other. You need to be clear with the student about what your expectations are, and to understand what hers are.

2. Responsibility conflicts: how much should the student do for herself and how much should you help, especially when you are busy and when the student is left with unstructured time?

3. Power differences: worries on the student's part that she may be penalised for acting independently or repeatedly seeking help.

4. Unshared meanings, particularly the inappropriate use of jargon.

The dynamics and impact of working groups upon students cannot be exaggerated. Difficult dynamics, misunderstood compliance and poor socialisation can all have a direct impact upon the care that is given. These factors will also adversely affect team spirit, successful group work and the pleasure of being a team member. The basics of supervision and mentorship cannot be overstated as powerful tools for achieving a strong and healthy culture.

KEEPING THE STUDENT BUSY

This section lists some activities that students can engage in to promote their learning. They must be linked to the learning outcomes that the placement hopes to achieve. You can either prepare these activities yourself or ask current students on the ward to help you prepare them. However, such activities do not substitute for talking and listening to students and interpreting the activities with them.

Work study analysis

A good teaching tool, and one you can use when you are busy, is to ask your student(s) to undertake an analysis of your work activity using a simple work study analysis sheet. Have two columns for the student to record what you are doing at regular intervals – perhaps every 15 minutes – and what she is doing. This should give you some fruitful material to analyse together, and should also help you when discussing your work in performance review or evaluating the way you work yourself.

There is limited literature in the UK available on systematic work study analysis. A work study may be constrained by recording only what is being done, rather than capturing the thoughts and interactive processes underlying the actions being recorded. The Royal College of Nursing (1996) suggests that it is impossible to capture the invisible (tacit) aspects of care that are more than just 'doing'.

Empirical and tacit skills also define the role of the registered nurse, but present a challenge to measure (Ford et al. 1997). To develop an accurate profile of activity, work sampling is most effective when carried out over a period of time and preferably on different shifts, so that you can draw up a rounded picture. For example, your activity on a theatre operating day would be very different to working a weekend.

Work sampling is a method that relies on the laws of probability. Observations taken at repeated random intervals will have the same distribution (Urden and Roode 1997). In this process, the exact activity is recorded but the time spent on the activity is not. Interrater reliability is an important factor in this method, so it is important to ensure that if several of you are doing this (or helping students to do it) you all agree on the definition and scope of the activity, so that you are all looking at the same thing. This method is useful for high-variability jobs, such as working with outpatients, moving from day-shift to night-shift, and so on, as observations can be translated into percentages of time spent in actual activities.

Activities are classified using a mutually exhaustive and exclusive list of all work categories. A large volume of observations need to be completed in order to have sufficient data for analysis if you are thinking about implications for the workforce, but if you are interested in analysing your own work patterns you may just want to analyse and compare a couple of shifts when you and your student are working together.

The complexity of nurse–patient relationships may not be captured by work analysis. Urden and Roode (1997) had three assumptions:

1. Nursing care is complex and involves critical thinking, ongoing assessment and evaluation throughout the direct and non-direct care-giving phase.

2. Many thought processes and interventions may occur at any one time during the care episode.

3. These processes are not captured in work sampling.

Urden and Roode went on to design a data collection instrument with five categories:

1. Direct care: all nursing care activities performed in the presence of the patient and family, assessing patients' needs, medicines, treatments, observations, specimens, basic physical care, communication, planning care, teaching, intervening and evaluating

2. Indirect care: all nursing care activities away from the patient but on the patient's behalf, communication with other providers, giving

reports, seeking consultation, preparing equipment, gathering supplies, preparing medicines

3. Unit-related: general maintenance (i.e. not patient-specific), clerical work, cleaning, ordering supplies, checking equipment, meetings, errands

4. Personal: not patient care or unit-related, meal breaks, adjusting personal schedules, personal phone calls, socialising with co-workers

5. Documentation: all activities to do with reviewing or evaluating patient care and condition.

You may have noticed that teaching and supporting students is not a category, and may wish to add this as a separate item.

Data collection consists of 4-hour time blocks for research and workforce purposes, but you may wish to reduce these to more manageable time chunks using boxes for the time of observation and code for the activity. In addition, you may want to record what the student is doing at the time, from passive observation to giving care.

Work sampling using the Urden and Roode (1997) process will, although time-consuming, give an accurate profile of exactly what nurses do, provide a medium for discussion with your student(s) and facilitate your reflections about how you and the nursing team work.

If the student records her own activity at the time, you can get a measure of what and how much she is learning, what she has perceived, any issues she has misunderstood and what she may wish to emulate. This will give the student something to do when you are working under pressure and are not able to devote the time that you feel you should to the student.

Recording your work activities will allow you to determine how much time you spend on non-nursing duties, and ascertain whether you are making best use of your expertise and experience. In many work studies, some tasks undertaken by registered nurses were not directly related to patient care, and so healthcare assistants could undertake these roles (Crouch 1992). One report stated that 60% of a nurse's time in this study was spent on non-nursing duties (Blay et al. 2002).

One criticism of work study analysis is that defining nursing as a series of interventions that can be observed and counted is reductionist, and does not account for the complexity of nursing care and the nature of clinical judgement. In other words, the analysis may reveal the quantity but not quality of care (Spilsbury and Mayhew 2001). The number of times that a task is performed may have no bearing on the quality of care that the patient receives (Gibbings 1995).

However, work sampling can give your students a purpose when their time is unstructured. It provides a powerful medium for discussion and support since students are able to question, challenge and reflect as they discuss what you and they did together. You could look at the work you did that matched the skills and insights that the student wanted to learn. From this, you may wish to plan with your student any activities that she can do unsupervised on your next shift together, where some supervised practice is needed, and where the student will rely on you to demonstrate the skill she is hoping to acquire.

If the student knows you are busy, she may feel under pressure not to delay you but then may be concerned about how she is going to meet her learning needs (Cooper 2001). This paper goes on to point out that students often feel uncomfortable in their observational role, and are keen to get on with giving care.

Cooper also identified that students found it difficult to articulate their learning needs on clinical placement, particularly if they lacked confidence and found objectives difficult to formulate. A period of work study analysis may create the medium for this, so that the student can understand how you work and where she can fit in.

This exercise will give the student something to do while you are busy. It will yield insight into the way that you both work and furnish plenty of material for reflection.

There may still be times in the shift when your priority has to be other than the student, leaving her at a loose end. You may recall from your own student days that there is nothing more deskilling than standing around not knowing what to do when everyone else looks focused and busy. Under these circumstances it may be worth devising some materials that the student can engage with independently. This will take the pressure off both of you, and still ensure that there are good learning opportunities to be taken up.

Learning contracts

A learning contract can be a useful tool to support student-centred, independent study and learning. It is simply a written agreement between mentor and mentee which makes explicit what the student will do to achieve specific learning outcomes. Nicklin and Kenworthy (2002) describe how a contract can help you to:

- Identify individual learning needs
- Set objectives to achieve outcomes
- Place an emphasis upon student activity
- Emphasise student–teacher interaction, and the subject matter and opportunities to be explored
- Promote teaching and learning by discovery
- Increase student motivation
- Individualise learning
- Promote adult learning.

These are all exemplary reasons for developing a learning contract, but it has to be delivered by yourself and the student – it is useless if just filed in a drawer. The student may also need considerable support to negotiate her needs, and to fulfil her side of the contract. Part of the process may be to explore the support mechanisms that are available to help the student to achieve fitness to practise.

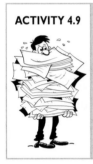

ACTIVITY 4.9

Take time with your student to devise a contract. You may also wish to do the same with your mentor. Are there things you want to develop where you are both going to play a part? If so, note the timescale and how your objectives will be measured and evaluated against the eventual outcome.

Patient pathways

Pollard and Hibbert (2004) describe how student-centred learning can be developed using patient pathways. These simply follow the patient's journey from referral for assessment, through to your clinical area, and then to follow-up and aftercare. This forms a sequence of learning events for the student, and may include pre-admission assessment in outpatients with diagnostic tests and procedures, visits with health professionals, such as the physiotherapist or radiographer, or observation in theatre.

This all makes it possible for a student to understand better what is happening to the patient, and get a complete picture. Patient pathways can thus provide a powerful medium for learning.

Consider designing some pathways for patients that the student can use with a learning diary or journal, so that she has a chance to reflect upon her perceptions with you at various stages in her experience.

You may be able to map pathways against the learning outcomes or competencies that you specified earlier for the student, so that her experience can be made directly relevant. The pathway may look like a worksheet with contact numbers and names for the student to sort her time and tasks. This negates the need to follow one patient through from admission to discharge (a task made more difficult by rapid patient throughput), and ensures that the student can fill in any gaps in her experience. The Pollard and Hibbert article (see above) is an enjoyable and thought-provoking read, and will give you some clear guidance on how to design student learning around patient pathways.

The 'world model'

Channel (2002) discusses the problems of mentoring students when there are staff shortages, an increasing volume of work and demands made by the growing complexity of care. The so-called world model outlined by Channel can be applied to any clinical setting using the following principles:

- A rota indicates which activities a student is undertaking during the week.
- Activities are negotiated with the student to meet learning needs.
- The rota can be planned in advance.
- The learning activities can be colour-coded so that each student can clearly identify what she should be doing and when.

The activities are:

- Working clinically: what skills need to be developed and who will supervise the process
- Observing experts, then using reflective practice to consolidate the observations
- Researching a topic: develop some cards so that the student is guided as to what to search for, prompted about where to look and what to do with the identified material, using the library to research care linked to practice
- Learning packs, which can be developed in advance
- Departmental visits.

All of these can be incorporated into your student learning contract, so that she can use her own initiative to structure her time purposefully with increasing independence and linked to the expected learning outcomes.

Patient satisfaction

The student may wish to take account of, and learn from, the patient's perceptions of experience in your care.

If work study analysis reveals what nurses do, patient satisfaction studies will reveal perceptions of quality of care which can be compared and contrasted to the findings of work sampling for the student. This means you have a record of what you both did and what the patient thought of it.

The Newcastle Satisfaction with Nursing Scale (an undated internet resource) is based on a six-point scale that focuses upon:

1. The provision of information
2. Empathy with the patient

3. Attitude to patient

4. Access to and continuity of the caregiver

5. Technical quality and competence

6. Overall satisfaction.

Data are collected from individual patients, but the tool has been developed for analysis at ward or clinic level rather than at patient level. It can be used to compare groups of patients at different points in time, or in different wards and clinics.

The document is available to download from http://www.ncl.ac.uk/chsr/publications/tools/nsnqst.doc. The scale is adaptable so that questions not relevant to your clinical area can be deleted, and additional questions inserted. The tool has been tested and validated as it is now, and not after adaptation. It gives details of sample size, how to administer the Statistical Package for Social Sciences (SPSS), ethical guidelines and methods of analysis. It is a ready-made package that can be tailored to meet the needs of yourself and your student, so that you can talk with the student about what happened to the patient as part of the student's observations and reactions.

Sections of the questionnaire can be used at different times. For instance, there is a section for the ward at night which could be used to reflect upon your night shift with your student. So you can either take sections of the questionnaire or do the whole thing. The researchers are suggesting a large sample size but you may only want to ask the patients you are currently caring for with the student.

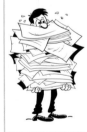

ACTIVITY 4.10

Take stock of what you have achieved so far for your own profile:

- Think about who you have chosen as your own mentor. Note the activities/behaviours that he or she undertakes that help you, such as the ability to listen and summarise
- Note the materials that you have ready for the student to start
- Write a note about the culture you work in and its strengths
- Record the activities that you have put in place to foster independent learning on the student's part and the skills you have used in developing these.

WORKING WITH THE STUDENT IN A PROFESSIONAL RELATIONSHIP

This section explores the phases of the mentoring relationship, and looks at how to start and end your work with your mentor and your mentee. It briefly describes a solution-focused way of communication (a useful skill for all walks of life), and then looks at different strategies for helping and analysing interactions. The potential for your skills development is enormous, providing a rich opportunity to observe the skills of your mentor as a role model as you develop your own.

There is no standard definition of a mentor, but mentoring can be accurately described as a two-way partnership between people. It is based on continuing support and development, tackling the needs, issues and blockages identified by the mentee and providing learning opportunities for both mentee and mentor. The Modernisation Agency Leadership Centre (2004) states that a mentoring relationship can be one of the most powerful developmental experiences that one will ever have. The Agency states that four out of five chief executives identify that having a mentor was one of their keys to success.

But you don't have to be an aspiring chief executive to benefit from this opportunity to develop others. We can probably all remember significant people who have profoundly influenced us and helped to fashion the ways we work.

The key to significant personalised learning is, then, a developmental relationship with someone of substantially greater experience who has taken a direct interest in you. Many of us in mentoring roles become anxious about the validity of our experience as one of the criteria for mentoring. This is especially true when our students have access to an evidence-base that we may not have encountered, or to knowledge that was not transmitted when we were learning nursing. However, even a nurse who has been qualified for a year has 4 years of experience that our novice mentees do not have, which should improve the nurse's perception of his or her role as mentor. Where the mentor can successfully interchange the role of teacher and learner, his or her students can help him or her to learn too – it is not a crime to admit we don't know something, but it is a crime to admit ignorance and then fail to remedy it. So a good mentor encourages a two-way flow of learning with the mentee.

A mentor may draw upon the skills of coaching, teaching and counselling to build up the capacity of the mentee, to help her discover her own wisdom, and to encourage the student to develop her own goals by forming a close working relationship.

Your mentee's needs will change as you help her in the transition from student to registered nurse. This must be the main purpose of your mentoring role.

Suen and Chow (2001) argue that mentoring is the most favoured model for managing student learning. Students with a mentor are more likely to receive planned and meaningful learning. Mentors ensure that students are supported in the clinical area.

Burns and Patterson (2005) suggest that mentoring has a direct effect upon the types of activity that students engage in while on clinical practice.

If the mentor failed to negotiate the learning role of the student with the ward team the student was often left to work with unqualified staff when the mentor was off-duty. The advocacy role of the mentor is a strong and powerful element in student learning.

The role of the mentor has been defined in numerous articles and chapters (Nicklin and Kenworthy 2002). There are some common principles emerging from the literature, for example that mentors teach from experience and by example (coaching); they use skills of facilitation, support and assistance to help students develop; and they create an experience that moves from mentor-centred to student-centred activity as the learning experience proceeds.

Empowering the student helps her to think critically about the nursing environment and her practice, and to develop her own body of knowledge.

Burns and Paterson (2005) identify many helping activities that mentors adopt:

- Engaging with the student in practice, challenging and following issues through, especially the tough ones
- Exploring alternative strategies for care, and opening up a range of options
- Promoting the personal and professional development of the student in line with the expectations and the requirements of the course
- Acting as professional role models
- Developing educational packages
- Ensuring the student receives supervision
- Identifying learning opportunities for the student
- Providing the student with ongoing formative assessment of the competencies she is expected to receive
- Summatively assessing the student
- Engaging in lifelong learning
- Evaluating one's own mentorship activities
- Evaluating the practice placement as a learning environment.

In addition, a mentor can discuss informally with his or her student apparent differences between theoretical knowledge and practice, relating this analysis to patient care.

There is some debate on whether it is appropriate for mentors to assess their mentees, and practice on this varies between the different partner universities. Mentees' commitments include:

- Willingness to be stretched and challenged (as well as supported) in achieving their personal goals

- Perceiving the value of tapping into someone else's different and wider experience
- Being prepared to acquire new learning
- Wanting to develop a whole range of additional learning resources for themselves, and exploring in full what your area has to contribute to this
- Developing their own goals and understanding what strengths they have in contributing to them
- Thinking about their expectations of you and themselves
- Taking responsibility in managing the relationship, for example by arranging meetings and setting the agenda to meet their needs. This is a skill that takes time and would benefit from some positive encouragement from you
- Showing consideration for your time, energy and emotions when things are difficult and challenging for you
- Demonstrating commitment by preparing for sessions with you, and carrying out agreed actions
- Being open and honest, listening to your views, accepting challenges and making up their own mind about what to do. They must also look after you and meet your needs in a reciprocal relationship, give you sensitive considered feedback about the nature and quality of the help you are giving them, and have a nurturing rapport.

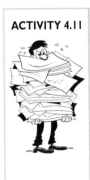

ACTIVITY 4.11

Return to the table in Activity 4.2. Under the box headed 'Demonstrating mentoring and facilitation skills', explore your skills and practice in each of the areas detailed by Burns and Paterson (2005), adding in the helping themes they identify as subheadings.

Develop your personal statement to reflect your skills. Give examples of how you encouraged critical thinking. Share this with your mentor, and discuss how to move forward in your strong areas and where you wish to improve your skill or knowledge.

So you may now have a sentence that reflects your ability to question and help students make links from their theoretical knowledge to practical care and be noting that you are keen to develop the skill of assessment.

Mentor–Mentee relationships

As mentor, you must be able to form a professional relationship with your students.

The Modernisation Agency Leadership Centre (2004) identifies five stages of mentoring, setting out guidance on how to manage your role and relationship with the student: (1) building rapport; (2) setting direction; (3) making regular progress; (4) winding up; and (5) moving on.

Building rapport

You have to decide if the personal chemistry between you and your prospective mentee is right or not. You may wish to check out your common ground, interests and beliefs, and what any differences are. This phase consists of negotiating how the relationship will be conducted and your mutual expectations.

If it appears that there is a lack of rapport, you need to be honest about the issues involved. You might have to agree to take a professional attitude to making the relationship work (recognising the differences between you), or find someone who can meet the student's needs better.

Key elements of rapport-building include:

- Trust: you both maintain confidentiality and keep your promises
- Focus: are you listening actively to your mentee? Are you open and non-judgemental?
- Empathy: respecting and understanding the other's point of view
- Congruence: a shared sense of purpose in the relationship, and an ability to share your own fears, weaknesses and mistakes
- Empowerment: encouraging your mentee to walk and then fly.

Good rapport can be measured by your body language (are you both comfortable?), whether you can explore difficult issues together without embarrassment, the quality of your discussions and a shared enthusiasm for learning.

The most important element of rapport-building is trust. The Modernisation Agency Leadership Centre (2004) identifies the core elements of trust as:

- Goodwill and a sense of caring
- Reliability (doing what you say you will do)
- Consistency and predictability
- Competence (you know what you are doing)
- Reciprocity (you listen to and respect others)
- Equity (treating people fairly).

ACTIVITY 4.12

FOR YOU AND YOUR MENTEE, AND FOR YOU AND YOUR MENTOR

Plan your first meetings with your student and mentor so that you begin to build rapport. Think about what expectations and hopes you have for the relationship, and what personal interests and stories you might share to establish common ground.

How did you demonstrate trust? Compare your student meeting with your first meeting with your mentor. How did your mentor build rapport, and why did you feel trusted? Compare and contrast the two approaches. Note anything that your mentor did that you will adopt in the future.

Include in your plan items such as how meetings will be organised; how you will ensure confidentiality; the professional boundaries governing reasonable behaviour and any areas not to be discussed; and how you will review progress as the relationship develops.

Plan for what happens if things don't work out between you. You might want to involve the university placement/practice facilitator or lecturer to help start off your plan, or (if necessary) involve this person if you and your mentee need to look at what is going wrong and what needs to be done. You may also need to discuss these issues with your own mentor.

Setting direction

This phase is where clear goals are developed to give the mentee a sense of direction and purpose. For the mentee, setting direction is about what you want to become, what will be different about you or your circumstances in a year's time, and how you will know you have made progress. The mentee needs to know what specific help the mentor will give her to achieve this.

The plan must focus on the learning outcomes of the placement, and define the student's priorities and actions the student must take to demonstrate she has acquired the necessary competencies.

There is a useful acronym for action-planning: SMART (specific, measurable, achievable, realistic, time-limited). This covers what you want to happen, how it will be measured, considers if it is achievable and realistic, and what time limit you are going to put on it.

You should prepare ahead for this, thinking about what is essential and what is desirable. Think about any areas in your knowledge that you may need to brush up, and identify issues for you and your mentee to resolve early. You should always be flexible in your approach even after years of mentoring, since every student is different.

Making regular progress

This is where most of your time and energy as mentor will be expended. You will use a wide range of skills to ensure your mentee's progress. These may include demonstrations of technique and practice, role-modelling, making introductions, lobbying for your student, encouraging her to network, offering firmness and clear guidance when things go wrong, and giving feedback on her learning and practice.

You should always keep your own log of your student's progress. If she intends to write (as she should) a reflective account of the placement, you might want to ask her for a copy of it to help you write your own log. Both of you will find your notes are essential to record progress, frustrations, obstacles, celebrations, learning points, differences of opinion, and so on.

Good preparation is called for, by both of you, for your regular meetings. Set up your meetings schedule and ensure that your student has a copy. Set the agenda in advance of each meeting. This should always include a review of your action plan and how it is being implemented, amending it if needed.

Never allow the relationship to deteriorate, for example by forgetting meetings, last-minute cancellations or struggling to give purpose to your dialogue with your student.

Winding up

In this phase, your student should have become more self-reliant and confident. She should now be setting the agenda and have become increasingly independent of you as mentor. Your working relationship should by now be firmly established, as your shared objectives should be achieved and you should have real confidence in each other.

The Modernisation Agency Leadership Centre (2004) identifies the risk that the relationship may cross boundaries here by moving into a counselling role, rather than just ending. If that were to happen, the student might become overly dependent on you for emotional support rather than for your continued professional development. This in turn can lead to feelings of guilt, resentment and so on.

Plan carefully for this end stage of mentoring. Both of you should summarise what you have learned and experienced. Discuss and plan for who will take your place as mentor. Don't allow your positive working 'helping' relationship to fade away without celebrating its success and learning from it.

Moving on

The relationship will now end, or in some cases grow into a personal friendship. With your own mentor, you may find that you continue to work together on a different action plan that enhances other aspects of your portfolio.

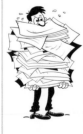

ACTIVITY 4.13

- Plan the structure of the meeting with your student. Summarise both your achievements and celebrate them
- After the meeting, reflect on the student's feedback to you. How did the meeting go? Think about how you are feeling. Is there anything you would change for future 'moving-on' meetings?
- Discuss this at your next meeting with your own mentor. Reflect on any issues (good or bad) that you have identified. What have you enjoyed in your role as mentor (or mentee)? What has frustrated you? What strengths have you developed? What new things have you learned? What advice would you now feel able to give to someone who is about to become a mentor or mentee for the first time?

COMMUNICATION AND MENTORING

Communication (the crux of mentoring) is a complex and demanding activity. Good communication requires paying attention, using active listening skills, monitoring the reactions of others, understanding both the content of what the other person says and any underlying non-verbal implications, responding in a way which confirms you have understood the message, and so on.

Communication has the following functions (Williams 2002):

- Giving information
- Seeking information
- Expressing emotions
- Communicating attitudes
- Establishing and maintaining relationships
- Regulating social interaction.

Northouse and Northouse (1998) describe how interprofessional communication consists of three elements: (1) the content of the message; (2) the relationship between the parties involved in the interaction; and (3) the context or setting in which the communication takes place.

A message with the same content will be very different if you ask a nurse to get intravenous fluids as part of a planned care programme, or if it is part of an urgent response to a patient collapse.

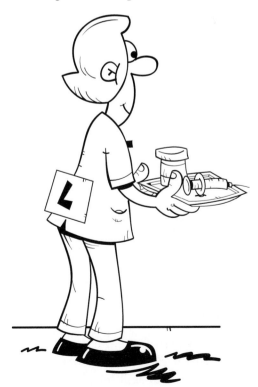

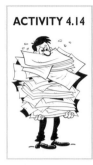

ACTIVITY 4.14

Ask your student to work with you during an episode of care to consider how you both demonstrated to the patient:

- Empathy: the ability to demonstrate to patients that you understand their feelings
- Trust: accepting the patient without judging
- Encouraging personal control
- Self-disclosure: the communication of personal information, thoughts or feelings
- Confirmation: making the patient feel worthwhile.

Solution-focused brief therapy (SFBT)

SFBT is a type of therapy first developed as family therapy (Dickson et al. 2001), but it is a useful style to adopt in everyday interaction.

The principles of SFBT require talking positively to colleagues you are supporting, as well as to clients. The therapy recognises that whatever the problem there will always be times when it is less severe, or even not present at all. Focusing on these times can make the person feel less overwhelmed by the problem. Take, for example, a student who fears watching patients being anaesthetised, or seeing a patient having a cardiac arrest. The student may feel quite unable to cope. But you may be able to identify aspects of (for instance) the patient's resuscitation in which the student is competent, can play a useful role and start to achieve confidence.

Identifying the person's preferred outcome for the problem is vital – that is, how she would like things to be. If you know this, it makes it much more likely that you can successfully communicate with her and try to resolve problems about the clinical experience. Take a nurse who is anxious when patients are undergoing anaesthetic induction. The solution for her problem will depend on whether she has any intention of ever having a career in a surgical environment, or if she wants to specialise in theatre or surgical care.

Key factors in solution-focused talking include:

- Focus on the person with the problem, rather than the problem in isolation
- Highlight the student's strengths and resources and what the student can do, rather than what she cannot do
- Discuss and consider what the student's preferred future would be in terms of learning and practice
- Discuss what may already be contributing to, or impeding, that preferred future
- Treat the student as a person who knows what is best for herself.

For each of these key factors, you can substitute 'patient' for 'student'. SFBF is a useful skill for all areas of life. Its emphasis on the positive and the need to minimise negative aspects is often self-fulfilling: if you expect positive things to happen, they will, but if you dismiss a student as hopeless she may behave in a way that reinforces your verdict on her. Focusing on the positive builds confidence and helps to promote success.

The main characteristic of a conversation with your student (or patient) when you are using SFBT is that your conversation will be solution-talk rather than problem-talk. For example:

- Problem-free talk: you listen to what the person's problem is, but do not dwell on it. You do not trivialise the problem: you need to understand it in order to help. You check what you really need to know before you ask the next question.

- Problem definition: ask the person to say what the problem actually is and how she feels you can help. Focus on what the person actually wants rather than what you think she wants. Be prepared to compromise, that is, you need to establish her preferred way of thinking and feeling rather than impose your ideal solution on her.

- Discuss what can be done to make this preferred future happen. What can the person already do? What can you do to help her achieve her objective? What are the steps or stages that represent progress towards this goal?

- Solution-talk: focus on the positive. This does not mean you ignore the person's distress or anxiety, but it does mean that you focus on the positive side – for example, how she has coped with it – rather than dwelling on intangible fears.

- Exceptions: when might things be easier, for example, practising a procedure when there are no doctors or medical students milling around.

- Finally, rate the student's responses to questions on a scale of 1–10. How might things feel in this or that scenario? How did she feel when she first saw something being done, and how does she feel now about that same thing? Can you plan some appropriate strategy for resolving any remaining problems?

ACTIVITY 4.15

Using solution-focused brief therapy (SFBT), talk to a student about one of the objectives she wishes to achieve on the ward. With her permission, tape-record (say for 5 minutes) your conversation with her. Transcribe the tape into different headings (what you said, what she said). In the third column, identify the SFBT strategies you used.

You will then have another skill to add to your profile.

You said	She said	Strategy used
Tell me a bit more about what is difficult	I find it hard to use the forceps and keep fumbling and contaminating them	Problem exploration

Framework for dealing with communication

John Heron (2001) proposed a communication framework called 'six-category intervention'. He suggests that you can categorise all your interventions with a client as follows:

1. Prescriptive

2. Informative

3. Confrontational

4. Cathartic

5. Catalytic

6. Supportive.

This six-category system represents the approach a professional might use when dealing with a client. Although the system resembles a counselling model, it applies just as well to students and patients. It is a useful way of analysing and reflecting upon the helpfulness of our interventions. It may assist you in raising your own awareness of what you want to achieve, and to consider alternative options if you cannot easily do this.

The six categories fall into two overarching headings as follows: (1) authoritative; and (2) facilitative.

Authoritative

- Prescriptive: the intervention aims to direct the behaviour of the student. You may instruct the student to do an action when you are at the bedside giving care.

- Informative: this aims to provide knowledge or information.

- Confronting: this aims to raise the student's awareness about some sort of attitude or behaviour which is jeopardising her success and of which she may be unaware.

Facilitative

- Cathartic: this aims to enable the student to show emotions like grief or fear.

- Catalytic: this aims to encourage the student to problem-solve and learn for herself.

- Supportive: this aims to affirm the value of the student, and to focus upon what she does well.

If you are too prescriptive, the student may not learn unless you explain the rationale for your action, perhaps later. For instance, dealing with a clinical emergency is not the time to draw a diagram of the heart and explain why adrenaline will help it to pump.

If you have to confront a student, find the right setting to do it, give examples of the negative behaviour, and then offer options that she could adopt to avoid such behaviour in future. Don't confront anyone unless you can also offer support, except of course in disciplinary procedures where different codes of conduct apply.

A cathartic intervention needs to take place in a safe environment so that emotion can be expressed and managed. Catalytic interventions and support are highly recommended as adult strategies to help others.

When did you last receive praise during feedback? If you can recall an instance, think about how you felt. As with confrontation, remembering your emotions will reinforce positive behaviour and help develop self-awareness.

There is nothing mystical about SFBT or Heron's six categories, since they are things we do every day (although in a practical non-theoretical fashion). This chapter is not intended to teach you communication

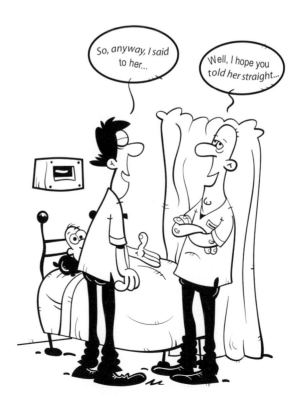

and counselling skills, but to remind you that they are at the heart of mentoring relationships and will help you to be aware of your support strategies.

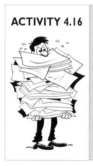

ACTIVITY 4.16

Return to your tape-recorded and transcribed record of your conversation with your student. Note when you used Heron's six categories, and whether they worked. Talk about this with your mentor or other support person and set some goals for your development, such as raising awareness of how you communicate. Write a paragraph for your portfolio on your communication style.

Reflective practice

Guidance by and support from your facilitator are essential to achieve meaningful reflective practice, because you do not want to mull over your experience in a purposeless fashion.

Without a structured process for reflection, it is easy to draw erroneous, inaccurate or meaningless conclusions. Using reflective techniques is a skill we all have to practise and develop. Reflection can be particularly helpful in encouraging nurses to write or discuss accounts of significant clinical experiences, to facilitate learning or provide an effective debrief for their colleagues. Written accounts are most useful to allow the nurse and others to evaluate what was perceived to happen, and what actually happened, and to learn from this.

A useful model of reflection was described by Gibbs and Pearce (2003). The model poses a series of questions which link into action and feedback:

- Description: what happened?
- Feelings: what were you thinking and feeling?
- Evaluation: what was good and/or bad about the experience?
- Analysis: what sense can you make of the situation?
- Conclusion: what else could you have done?
- Action plan: if you were to do it again, what would you change?

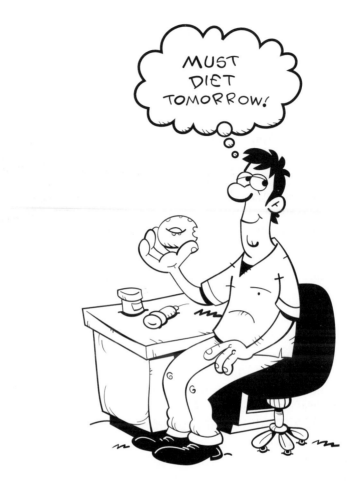

There are many reflective models which are available for use, but they all look at what actually happened, they ask you to describe the feelings associated with the event, and then move on to evaluating the outcomes or options which were not, in the end, exercised. Reflection can occur during an experience, when you might say: 'Let's stop for a moment to think about alternative actions and their likely outcomes'. Or reflection can, of course, take place after an episode of care or client interaction. In either case, new understandings should emerge for application to the next relevant situation.

Giving students feedback

Giving students accurate and timely feedback is critical to their personal and professional development, and to promoting their self-awareness as nurses.

Remember the last time you had feedback from someone that really helped you in your work? This may not have happened frequently. Think about what the feedback was. Did it focus upon one of your strengths, or was it relevant to an area you could improve? Now, think about the context of the feedback, the mood you were in, and what you took away from the experience. If the roles were reversed and you were giving the feedback, what would you repeat and what would you do differently?

In professional life, the main – if not only – reason for giving feedback is to help. You should not give feedback if your real motivation is to hurt or confuse the other person. You give feedback on performance to achieve or reinforce positive aspects of behaviour.

One beneficial consequence of positive feedback is to raise the recipient's self-esteem. Positive feedback motivates people to do even better. It reinforces positive behaviour, and makes colleagues who may be feeling vulnerable and anxious realise that you approve of them. A lack of feedback will leave your student feeling confused, out of place, and unsure of whether she 'fits into' the group. This in turn will generate anxiety and low self-esteem, and may unhelpfully cause the student to go into a negative-feedback loop, feeling uncomfortable and unvalued.

The timing of feedback is important. It is essential that you consider the student's needs, so (for example) if the student has made some mistake it may be important to stop or take over the patient procedure, but it would not be good to go into detail until the student is calm and over the shock. Generally, however, it is good to offer feedback as soon as you can after the student's performance, to encourage timely reflection – but not in front of the patient.

Do not give feedback if either you are, or the student is, upset or angry. Always consider the environment in which you offer feedback, and choose a place and time comfortable for you both, where you cannot be overheard.

When offering feedback, always concentrate on the student's strengths first. Discuss with the student how her strengths can be best applied in both the present and future. Quite often, students may need and value clear direction or advice on how to be even better at what they are good at, as much as they need advice on avoiding poor performance.

Always focus upon aspects of behaviour that you have directly observed. Do not rely on gossip, hearsay or unwarranted assumptions. If you wish to raise negative points with your student, consider carefully how to do this. We all find it easy to listen to praise, but most people find it difficult to accept critical feedback even when we accept that our performance may have called for such criticism.

If there are more than three issues of concern you wish to raise, try to group them into headings to avoid overwhelming the student. Prioritise that which matters the most. Are there things the student is doing which, if addressed, will solve other potential or actual problems?

End your feedback session with the most positive aspects of the student's performance, so that criticism is sandwiched between positive and supportive news.

Always make your feedback (whether on strengths or weaknesses) specific. It needs to be descriptive rather than evaluative, and objective rather than subjective. General and vague comments are of no use, since they may come across to the student as platitudes.

You should clearly describe the student's behaviour, by giving examples. Focus on any undesirable behaviours that can be changed, provided that you have a possible solution. For instance, someone's nervous cough may be very irritating, but if you do not know how to prevent her from coughing, it is not helpful to comment on it and can indeed make things worse.

This is particularly true when you are describing attitudes. Attitudes have three components – thinking, feeling and acting – which tend to go together. Changing undesirable attitudes can be problematic, but one tactic is to focus on one of the three components with a view to changing the others. For example, if a student seems very surly and distant when the doctors are on the ward, it would help to know what she is thinking and feeling. You may be able to alter what she is thinking by giving some information, making introductions or including the student in interactions. To change her behaviour, you may ask her to use open and accepting body language when this doctor is around, and then offer feedback to her on the difference it makes.

Good feedback will enhance the student's understanding, and encourage her to appreciate what works for her and how to alter the things that don't. Your own behaviour will, of course, influence the significance of your feedback. If the student feels you are interested in her, if you give time to explain and answer questions, if you are open and encouraging, if you praise and comment on her progress, if you are available, and especially if you show a sense of humour, this makes your feedback much more valuable. Were you able to identify any of these supportive behaviours in your own reflection?

Similarly, there are things you must never do if you wish to be effective in your feedback. Don't be threatening or 'scary' because the student will find it hard to listen to what you are saying. Sarcasm may make the student laugh with you at the time, but may secretly cause hurt. An attitude of superiority and making put-downs leave people unable to act as adults, as do making belittling comments, criticising or correcting in front of others.

Consider giving written feedback, by preparing a statement summarising how the student has done. Verbal offerings can be distorted or twisted by faulty memory, especially if someone is stressed or self-conscious. The written word is a permanent record of what you said, and is a powerful medium for reinforcing your message and assisting the student to assimilate and act upon it. There may be a form available for this from your partner university.

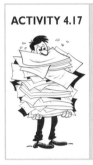

ACTIVITY 4.17

Write down the strengths you have learned and developed as a mentor. If necessary, return to Table 4.1 to prompt thinking on your part. Identify three areas which you would like to develop. Now write down what you think your greatest strength is.

Adapt the personal statement that you drew up at the start of this chapter for your profile. Consider whether your hopes and aspirations for yourself as a mentor and teacher have changed. Discuss this with your mentor as part of what you do next to promote development.

PREPARING TO LEARN FROM THE STUDENT PLACEMENT: CLOSING THE CIRCLE

Evaluation of the student placement: closing and cementing learning

Evaluation should not take place only at the end of the student's placement. You should consider evaluating a new task you have never done before, or carry out a routine evaluation at the end of the student's week. Evaluation can be done on a one-to-one basis, or with your group or team.

However and whenever you do an evaluation, explore with your student(s) your range of perspectives. Discuss your perceptions of what worked and what didn't. How, in the light of the evaluation, would you wish to do things differently?

You can start to identify gaps in learning. Return to your list of what the student *must* learn and what she *could* learn. Check out before the end of the placement if you need to ensure that all essential learning has been achieved and demonstrated where applicable. Once this primary objective has been realised, identify any other areas where the student could be encouraged to learn more.

The student may come with an already-made evaluation tool, or there may be a placement evaluation session in the university that you could attend. Discuss the student's perceptions with your placement facilitator and with your clinical team, making plans to build on her strengths and improve any areas where she did not achieve good performance.

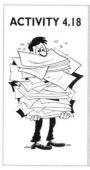

ACTIVITY 4.18

Reflect on your experience and triumphs in mentoring. What did you enjoy – and what did you not? What aspects of the experience would you repeat? What would you change? What needs to be developed? What is now 'off the shelf' and ready to use or adapt for the next placement student(s)? What new skills have you learned?

Have you, as a result of being mentored yourself, extended your professional network?

Of course, this list of questions is not exhaustive. Take time to think about these issues, ensuring that the teaching and mentoring side of your profile has been adapted to reflect your experiences.

CONCLUSION

This chapter has covered a number of ideas and theories to help you to support students in their work and placement. Some of the material will be familiar; some will serve as a reminder of what you already know; and some of it may have offered you new ideas and ways of working. In all cases, the skills of offering support grow as we develop. Teaching and learning is a dynamic process based on your knowledge and skills and ability to help others learn. You will remember the person or range of staff who helped you to learn and grow and now your students will reflect on your abilities in the same way. But even more than that, you will have made a difference to the care our patients receive.

Do not put that profile in the drawer. There is more to be developed as the next students arrive!

REFERENCES

Blay N, Cairns J, Chisholm J et al. (2002) Research into the workload and roles of oncology nurses within an outpatient oncology unit. European Journal of Oncology Nursing 6: 6–12

Burns I, Paterson I M (2005) Clinical practice and placement support: supporting learning in practice. Nurse Education in Practice 5: 3–99

Channel W (2002) Helping students to learn in the clinical environment. Nursing Times 98: 35–39

Coon D (1998) Introduction to psychology: exploration and application, 8th edn. Pacific Grove, California: Brooks/Cole

Cooper J M (2001) A student nurse's learning in a leg ulcer outpatient department. British Journal of Nursing 10: 150–161

Crouch R (1992) Technician, cleaner, clerk or nurse? Nursing Times 5: 30–32

Dickson D, Hargie O, Morrow N (2001) Communication skills training for health professionals. London: Chapman and Hall

Ford P, Heath H, McCormack B et al. (1997) What a difference a nurse makes. London: RCN

Fretwell J (1980) An inquiry into the ward learning environment. Nursing Times 76: 69–73

Gibbings S (1995) Dependency, skill mix, grade mix and their effects on health visiting practice. Journal of Clinical Nursing 4: 43–47

Gibbs M, Pearce R (2003) Profiles and portfolios of evidence. Cheltenham: Nelson Thornes

Hecht M, Jackson R, Pitts M (2005) Culture: intersection of intergroup identity theories. Intergroup communication: multiple perspectives. New York: Peter Lang

Heron J (2001) Helping the client: a practical guide. London: Sage

McBrien B (2006) Clinical teaching and support for learners in the practice environment. British Journal of Nursing 15: 672–677

Modernisation Agency Leadership Centre (2004) Leadership and race equality: mentoring programme. Burnham: Clutterbuck Associates

Moore S, Aiken D D, Chapman S (2005) Sociology. London: Collins

Nicklin P J, Kenworthy N (2002) Teaching and assessing in nursing practice: an experiential approach, 3rd edn. Lincoln: Tork

Northouse L, Northouse P (1998) Health communication strategies for health professionals, 3rd edn. London: Prentice Hall

Nursing and Midwifery Council (2008) The code: standards of conduct, performance and ethics for nurses and midwives. London: NMC

Pennington C (2004) Students need support. British Journal of Nursing 3: 1067

Pollard C, Hibbert C (2004) Expanding student learning using patient pathways. Nursing Standard 19: 40–43

Price B (2007) Practice-based assessment strategy for mentors. Nursing Standard 21: 49–56

Royal College of Nursing (1996) The values and skills of nurses working with older people. London: RCN

Spilsbury K, Mayhew J (2001) Defining the nursing contribution to patient outcomes: lessons from a review of the literature examining nursing outcomes skill mix and changing roles. Journal of Clinical Nursing 10: 13–14

Spouse J (2001) Workplace learning: pre-registration nursing students' perspectives. Nurse Education in Practice 1: 149–156

Suen L K P, Chow F L W (2001) Students' perceptions of the effectiveness of mentors in an undergraduate nursing programme in Hong Kong. Journal of Advanced Nursing 36: 505–511

Urden L, Roode J (1997) Work sampling: a decision-making tool for determining resources and work redesign. Journal of Nursing Administration 27: 34–41

Williams D (2002) Communication skills in practice. A practical guide for health professionals. London: Jessica Kingsley

Woodward W (2003) Preparing a new workforce. Nursing Administration Quarterly 23: 3

5	# How to assess teaching and learning

Dave Barton

INTRODUCTION

This chapter deals specifically with the theory and practice of educational assessment of learning. It will guide you through the foundation principles of this topic, and also take you on a brief tour of some commonly used assessment tools that you will encounter.

You may view the assessment of teaching and learning in a traditional way – as an outcome, as an end-point, as the fundamental activity of gauging the effectiveness and success of your teaching and of your students' learning activity. If that is the case you will need to change your view to a broader, and more practical, perspective of assessment of teaching and learning as a continuum, as a continual process that occurs constantly in education (and indeed throughout life). Thus, assessment is not just the end-point of any teaching and learning activity – it is the foundation of measuring and judging the need, process, progress, outcome and value of teaching in all areas of curriculum and learning.

LEARNING OBJECTIVES

By the end of this chapter you should be able to:

◆ Describe the essential difference between teaching and learning

◆ Explain and describe the different activity domains of teaching and learning

◆ Identify and describe the broad range of relevant assessment tools that you may encounter in practice

◆ Describe the principles of educational assessment

◆ Describe and explain an assessment strategy

◆ Identify specific assessment tools and:
  – explain how, why and where you use these assessment tools
  – explain how you prepare and support students for these assessments
  – explain how you prepare and support teachers and examiners for these assessments.

The chapter begins by exploring some key educational concepts and theoretical foundations that will assist you when first using the tools associated with assessment of teaching and learning. This is followed by examples and explanations of assessment tools that are commonly used in education. However, I must emphasise that this section does not cover every possible tool of assessment – to provide that would require an entire book of its own! Thus, the intention of this targeted sample of assessment tools is not only to illustrate how diverse they can be, but also to illustrate the common features and issues that arise for all such tools, and to give you transferable guidance on how such tools may best be designed and selected to meet the needs of your teaching. These examples are all structured and described by using the standard heading format:

● What is the assessment tool?

● What is the assessment tool testing?

● How valid is the assessment tool?

● How reliable is the assessment tool?

● What resource issues arise from this assessment tool?

● What other issues must be accounted for when using this assessment tool (regulations, professional requirements, safety, ethics, competence)?

● Preparation of the tool for use

● Preparation of examiners/assessors

● Preparation of students

● Marking and related issues

By using this standard structure I hope it will become clear that, whilst tools of assessment have many features in common, they can also be highly specific. Thus, although assessment tools may be used individually, they are also commonly used in groups (assessment strategies) that combine them together in varied ways to provide a wide-ranging and systematic foundation for assessing student development and performance. That being the case, completion of this chapter should provide you with the knowledge and skill to use assessment as a means of exploring not just assessment tools, but also wider curriculum issues, curriculum design and more encompassing learning strategies and outcomes.

Note that there are fundamental points raised in this chapter that are reviewed and explained elsewhere in this book, and you will benefit from reading all of the chapters in developing your wider understanding of assessment of learning.

ACTIVITY 5.1

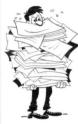

Take a few moments to think about and list the various educational assessments you have encountered throughout your life – whether as a student, as a teacher or in your clinical practice.

What was your impression of them? How did they affect you (were they useful as learning tools, or were they just hurdles to overcome)?

Although assessments of learning are something we all experience, they are unfortunately commonly viewed as stressful events, coloured by the fear of failure, and unsurprisingly related to issues of self-esteem, ambition and personal achievement. You have probably already noted in your list that you have had experience of assessments that made you anxious! Consequently it is crucial that the teacher acknowledges that assessment is always significant to students.

However, in professional healthcare education, assessment is also the gate of entry to a professional career – it affords the 'right to practise', and this makes the assessment process doubly stressful.

Thus, it is important to ensure that assessment of learning is educationally and professionally purposeful and useful, and that assessments do not become just hurdles that students have to overcome and which contribute little to their eventual practice or career.

ASSESSMENT – CONCEPTS, DEFINITIONS AND TERMINOLOGY

Chapter 3 has outlined a range of terms and definitions to aid your comprehension of educational vocabulary in relation to the use of competencies (Box 5.1). However, I will now add to this vocabulary exercise by considering some of the terms and definitions that relate specifically to education and assessment. This is necessary because, as with competencies, assessment and learning have a language of their own that you must understand if you are to use assessment effectively.

BOX 5.1	*The language of educational assessment*

Assessment

The act of judging or assessing a person, situation or event
- Assessment is about gathering information and data on performance
- Assessment is a qualitative process
- Assessment may be a diagnostic, formative, or summative exercise
- Assessment focuses on individuals

Assessment may be referenced by criterion (pre-established standard criteria or competencies)

Assessment may be referenced by norm (norm referencing measures or grades a student's performance achievement by reference to his or her peers' achievement and performance – this is useful as a developmental guide)

Evaluation

To ascertain or fix the value or worth of – examine, judge and carefully appraise
- Evaluation is about making a value judgement on the assessment information
- Evaluation is a quantitative process
- Evaluation is a summative exercise
- Evaluation focuses on concepts, groups or organisations
- Evaluation may be referenced by norm or criterion

Formative assessment (assessment for learning)

Ongoing and varied assessments which teachers and students use to gauge learning progression and identify (diagnose) problems or learning needs.
- Formative assessment provides students with feedback on their learning and helps their further development
- Formative assessment activities are important in motivating and enhancing learning
- Formative assessment activities can be diverse and are not included in the formal grading of work

Summative assessment (assessment of learning)

The formal testing of learning that produces marks or grades.
- Summative assessment has an evaluative component and may also be an employment, regulatory or legislative requirement
- Summative assessment is regarded as an end-point analysis of the extent and quality of learning – during or at the end of an educational course or module of learning
- Summative assessment may be undertaken using a wide range of assessment tools

Assessment tools (examples)
- Case history reports
- Clinical mentorship/supervision
- Portfolios (academic/clinical)
- Reflection (in practice – whilst you are doing it)
- Reflection (on practice – after you have done it)
- Practice diaries
- Competency frameworks
- Practical examinations
- Practical exercises (examiner-observed/written reports)
- Objective structured clinical examinations (OSCEs)

Other educational terms (see Table 3.2 in Chapter 3)
- Education
- Teaching
- Training
- Learning
- Curriculum
- Syllabus
- Mentor, supervisor, clinical teacher, preceptor
- Competence, competency

Assessment tools (examples) (Continued)
- Essays
- Dissertation (a lengthy written essay, treatise, or thesis – usually research-based)
- Project reports
- Written examinations (seen/unseen essays multiple choice questions (MCQs), short answers)
- Seminars/presentations
- Critiques (critical evaluation of literature)

To develop your understanding of assessment and learning fully, it is important that you realise that 'teaching' and 'learning' (although intimately linked), do not mean the same thing. In fact, to teach and to learn mean quite different things! Thus applying assessment tools to either has a different meaning and purpose. I have previously defined (Chapter 3, Box 3.2) teaching as the activity of educating or instructing: an activity that imparts knowledge or skill. In contrast I defined learning as a cognitive process of acquiring skill or knowledge that results in changed or new behaviour. Finally, assessment was defined as the act of judging or assessing a person or situation or event.

To understand these demands of assessment on education it is important that you draw these three terms together, that you compare and contrast them and consequently understand the tensions that exist between them.

Figure 5.1 illustrates how these commonly used educational terms of 'learning', 'teaching', and 'assessing' are all interlinked, and that the interaction between them brings many interesting and complex interpretations. Thus, although you may use these everyday terms with ease, you must also acknowledge the underlying meanings and complexity of relationships between them that will affect your use of assessment tools. For example, what aspect of learning or teaching are you trying to assess, what tools should you best use to undertake such assessment reliably and validly and – importantly – what will the assessment achieve?

Teaching and learning – activity domains and tools of assessment

Although I have explained that teaching and learning mean different things, they are for practical purposes grouped together into specific activity domains. In Box 5.2 I have presented those domains with examples of the teaching and learning activities that are commonly (but not necessarily exclusively) associated with them.

FIGURE 5.1 *Conceptual tensions – teaching/learning/assessment.*

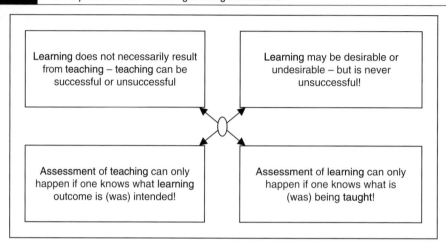

| BOX 5.2 | *Activity domains of teaching and learning* |

Teaching and learning: formal (traditional) learning – taught
- Being told (lessons, lectures, presentations)
- Being shown (examples, demonstrations)
- By observing (the lecturer, the clinical expert)
- By traditional studying (books, media)
- Through experiments (laboratories)
- Through simulations (practice suites, information technology, computer-assisted learning)

Teaching and learning: practice-based learning – experiential
- In practice (with clinical supervisors, mentors, preceptors – practice-based coaching, by imitation and through repetition of practice)
- By structured and reflective clinical supervision
- By diverse exposure to practice (direct experience and varied placements and clinical contact)
- By membership (working in a practice-based clinical team)
- In an apprenticeship (prolonged practice with one or more expert mentors or practitioners)

Teaching and learning: self-directed learning – personal and individual
- Through internet-based educational resources, computer-assisted learning, internet or traditional library resources, structured distance learning provision
- By asking
- Through public presentation
- By developing evidence-based personal concepts and relationships
- By having individualised (structured) motivation (aims)
- Through critical reflection

Teaching and learning: chance learning – serendipity
- In practice
- By teaching others
- Through trial and error
- By experiencing failure and success
- Through intuition and instinct (tacitly)

BOX 5.3   *Domains of learning – assessment tools*

Teaching and learning: formal (traditional) learning – taught
Often assessed by:
- Essays
- Project reports
- Dissertations (a lengthy written essay, treatise, or thesis – research-based)
- Written examinations (seen/unseen, essays, multiple choice questions, short answers)
- Seminar/presentation
- Critiques (critical evaluation of literature)
- Case history reports
- Reflection (in or on practice)
- Competency frameworks

Teaching and learning: practice-based learning – experiential
Often assessed by:
- Clinical mentorship/supervision
- Case history reports
- Project reports
- Practice portfolios
- Reflections (in or on practice)
- Diaries
- Competency frameworks
- Practical examinations
- Practical exercise (examiner-observed/ written reports)
- Objective structured clinical examination (OSCEs)

Teaching and learning: self-directed learning – personal and individual
Often assessed by:
- Reflections (in or on practice)
- Portfolios (academic/practice – clinical)
- Seminars/formal presentations
- Competency frameworks
- Project reports
- Portfolios (academic/clinical)

Teaching and learning: chance learning – serendipity
Often assessed by:
- Clinical mentorship/supervision
- Seminars/chance presentation
- Critique (critical evaluation of literature)
- Case history reports
- Reflection (in or on practice)
- Diaries/journals
- Competency frameworks

You will have noted that these learning and teaching activity domains are in practice closely interlinked, and that the boundaries between them are at best tentative. It is clear that some teaching and learning activities – and strategies – could apply to all domains. Thus, you should use Box 5.2 as a basic and *flexible* guide to the activity domains of learning and teaching.

These learning and teaching activity domains are also important to you as they are linked to the range and diversity of assessment tools available. Consequently the activity domains can guide you to the assessment tools that may best be selected for particular types (activities) of learning and teaching. In Box 5.3 I have listed the assessment tools that are most commonly associated with specific learning and teaching activity domains. However, I must again emphasise that there is no hard and fast rule that will preclude any assessment activity from any activity domain, and you will note that some assessment tools are associated with all activity domains.

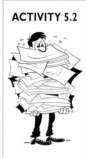

ACTIVITY 5.2

List the assessment tools that you commonly have seen or used in your area of practice.

Then consider the teaching and learning activity domains in Box 5.3. Write down how these apply, or do not apply, to your list of assessment tools – and how this then compares or contrasts with the range of assessment tools outlined in Box 5.4.

Do you think that assessment in your practice area is consistent with, or at odds with, local or national frameworks and competencies that are guiding your practice, e.g. *The NHS Knowledge and Skills Framework* (Department of Health 2004) and the *Guide to Advanced Practice* (Royal College of Nursing 2007).

Would you consider changing, or adding to, the assessments you are using? Remember, practice and education (and thus assessment) are constantly changing and evolving to meet new situations and demands – what was 'right' before may not be right today or tomorrow!

ASSESSMENT OF TEACHING AND LEARNING

Principles and outcomes of assessment

Assessment of teaching and learning should not be an arbitrary or random activity. If you wish to assess your students, you must also be able to justify and defend the assessment process. Assessment of teaching and learning must, therefore, be purposeful, productive and, above all, be based on sound and rational principles.

Checklist of assessment principles

- Assessment should motivate (not deter!).
- Assessment is a process that should be embedded in any teaching and learning activity.
- Assessment should serve an educational purpose (should benefit the student, assist the teacher, guide outcomes and measure performance).
- Assessment tools should promote and enhance quality education.
- Assessment tools should promote and enhance quality practice.
- Assessment may be identified by specific educational tools and strategies.
- Assessment tools should be rigorous and structured.
- Assessment strategies (combined multiple tools) should be rigorous and structured.
- Assessment should be objective.
- Assessment tools should be consistent and reliable.
- Assessment should be measurable and based on predetermined criteria.

- Assessment tools should be valid, i.e. meas~~ intended to measure.

- Assessment may be a diagnostic process.

- Assessment may be periodic, continuous or

- Assessment may be informal or formal.

- Assessment should channel outcome, but als

- Assessment may be a methodology for gauging individual or organisational ability and performance.

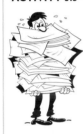

ACTIVITY 5.3

Consider the assessment principles above and use this checklist to examine an assessment tool (or tools) you have experienced or used.

How many points of the checklist agreed with your experience?

What did this tell you about the efficacy and rationale of the assessment strategy you considered?

It is easy to select an assessment tool for use – just pick one out of a list! It is however more difficult to ensure that an assessment tool is the right one. For example, it is relatively easy to set a written examination for a clinical skill such as manual handling, or administering intravenous drugs. You may get long, well-referenced and satisfactory answers to your questions – but what will this tell you about the student's actual practice skill when moving and handing clients, or when administering intravenous drugs? Thus, although the written exam has its place in testing the student's background knowledge of these skills, clinical mentorship or an objective structured clinical examination would be more useful in measuring his or her practical dexterity and fluency in enacting these skills.

Assessment strategies

It is clear from the principles above that assessment is a fundamental part of the structure and design of the teaching and learning process. Consequently the assessment tools that you select for your educational programmes or curriculum will have significant influence on *what* your students will learn, and *how* your students will learn. Thus, assessment forms a cornerstone of curriculum design and is not just concerned with marks and grades.

I have shown that different assessment tools may be suited to different learning outcomes, and so far I have generally referred to tools of assessment in the singular sense. However, programmes of education commonly have multiple learning outcomes, and these complicated curricula will draw not just on singular assessment tools, but will combine several or many tools, where each tool is testing specific outcomes. These combinations of assessment tools are referred to as 'assessment strategies'. In practice it is far more likely that you will be involved with educational programmes that will be using assessment strategies with multiple assessment tools (rather than just one individual assessment tool). Consequently, it is important for you to develop a broad understanding of the range and forms of assessment tools that you will encounter in practice, together with a sensible appreciation of the advantages and limitations of each. Your understanding of the rationale for the selection and combination of assessment tools within an assessment strategy is crucially important for you when later supporting, guiding and assessing students in practice.

Box 5.4 shows a simple example of an assessment strategy. This is drawn from a non-medical prescribing module run for professional nurses and pharmacists and other allied health professionals. Non-medical prescribing requires the practitioner to be numerically competent, knowledgeable in aspects of pharmacology and pathology, able physically to assess a patient proficiently, and capable of making diagnostic and clinical management decisions. It is clear that there is no one assessment tool that can in itself achieve this. Thus the curriculum/module designers have utilised several assessment tools – a combination of formal written examination, clinical portfolios and clinical practice exams (objective structured clinical examinations or OSCEs). The weighting of each tool contributes to the final grade, and a competency framework is employed to structure and map the eventual required competency outcome.

BOX 5.4	Example of an assessment strategy		
	Non-medical prescribing course Assessment strategy (example)	**Weighting (example)**	**Assessment strategy**
	Objective structured clinical examination (OSCE) examination	40%	OSCE assesses clinical assessment skills, diagnostic management skills and communication skills
	Practice (clinical) portfolio (content may be dictated or recommended, e.g. reflective accounts, case histories, video or audiotape analysis, competency checklists, mentor's verification)	30%	Portfolio assesses all areas of non-medical prescribing competency
	Multiple choice examination – pathology and pharmacology	30%	Multiple choice questions assess foundation knowledge of pathology and pharmacology
	Maths test	Pass/fail	Maths test assesses numeracy competence (although not included in to the final grade, the strategy requires the student to pass the maths test to be successful)

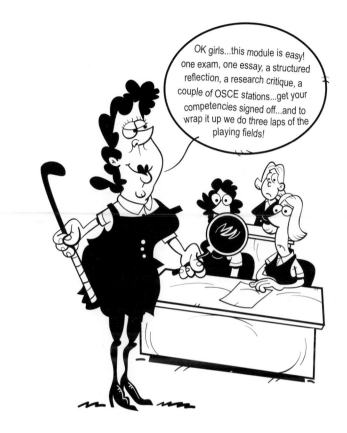

Student assessment and programme evaluation

In this section you need to consider in more detail two key issues that have already been touched on – why you assess students, and how assessment informs programmes of education. The first issue may be self-evident to the teacher in clinical practice but the role of assessment in programme evaluation may be less obvious initially. Thus, it is important that you understand that programmes of professional education are rooted in practice, dependent on practice resource, practice expertise and practice outcomes. Professional education is thus intimately linked to practice, and assessment outcomes are therefore inextricably related to programme performance.

Assessing students

At the most basic level you assess your students to establish four things:

1. Knowledge – what they know
2. Skill – what they can do
3. Performance – how well they do it
4. Motivation – their attitude – why they do it and how they feel about it.

These four principles provide a general guide and rationale for your preliminary selection of assessment tools. The subsequent design and refinement of the tools you have selected can be tested by asking standard questions. The answers to these questions will establish the reliability, validity and rigour of the assessment process you have designed.

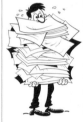

ACTIVITY 5.4

SELECTING, DESIGNING AND REFINING AN ASSESSMENT TOOL

Curriculum design is not a lone or individual activity. Well-constructed professional curricula and modules are designed by curriculum teams (committees) – these draw on wide-ranging academic and practice expertise. Experienced clinical educators are commonly asked to contribute to curriculum committees and as such it is important that you have a broad understanding of curriculum and assessment design. Although you may see yourself as primarily the user (mentor, examiner) of an assessment tool, you may also be party to its design, critique and subsequent refinement.

With that in mind, think of a learning outcome you would like to assess. Then answer the following questions:

- What is it that actually needs to be assessed?
- What is the minimum standard that could be expected from the student?
- What competencies could be used?
- What are the functions of the assessment? Is it diagnostic (telling you what the student needs to learn)? Is it formative (telling you how well the student is progressing)? Is it summative (telling you how well the student has achieved on completion)?

Once you can answer these questions your next step is to choose an appropriate instrument or method for assessment and consider its use in detail. Having selected an assessment tool, consider the following questions:

- Will this tool actually assess what needs to be assessed?
- What will be the marking criteria?
- Where will the assessment take place (in the classroom, or in practice)? Who should be involved in assessment (a lecturer, a clinical expert or practitioner, a mentor or even the student's peers)?
- What will I do with the result of the assessment? Is it part of a wider formal assessment strategy? Can the student fail? Can the student resit? Should it be used as an evaluative result for the teacher's performance? In addition, should it be available to, or used by, employers to judge the employee?

Remember that you must see the big picture! Students are commonly required to undertake many different forms of assessment, and you must be aware of the totality of the learning and assessment strategies if you are to support them in all their needs. Beyond that, you should be able to offer your expertise in evaluating and evolving assessment strategies as a result of your direct exposure to their application in practice.

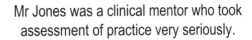

Mr Jones was a clinical mentor who took
assessment of practice very seriously.

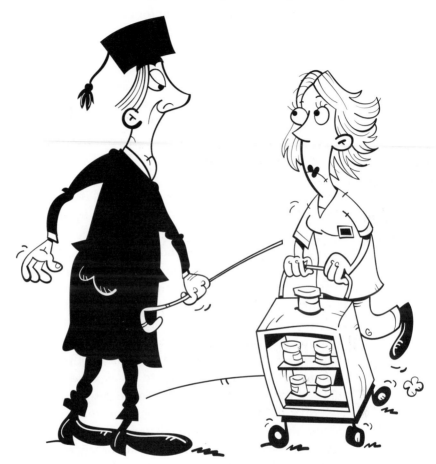

Programme evaluation

By now you should have no doubt that assessment is a key determinant of what
and how we teach. As assessment is so intrinsically bound up with the programme (course, scheme, module, plan) of education from which it arises, it
will also inevitably become one of the main mechanisms of programme evaluation. Programme evaluation may also be achieved by a wide variety of other
means (academic peer evaluation, student evaluation, attrition rates, multicentre
comparisons, expert user commentaries) – none of which will be explored here.

Assessment is a measure of student progression and practice outcomes;
it is also a key to the perceived value and success of a programme and to
decisions on programme modification and improvement. At a more focused

level, teachers will use assessment outcomes as a means of evaluating the success of their own teaching and the efficacy of their programme management – have they delivered what they set out to deliver, and are their students (and consequently the curriculum) fit for purpose?

There is no question that assessment statistics are used by government and commissioning bodies to judge educational institutions' performance and future funding. Equally, assessment strategies are subject to a range of validation and quality mechanisms from both within organisations and from wider audit authorities, as checks of progression, appropriateness, safety and outcome.

Assessment and the teacher

For the novice teacher it may at first seem that the process of assessment is a relatively simple matter of selecting assessment tools and getting students to complete them. By now you should be able to see that assessment is more complex than this; it is bound up with curriculum design, student experience and the relevance of the learned outcome. However, it is also important to understand that assessment has a fundamental and conceptual role to play in your understanding of your own skills and practice as a teacher.

To assess effectively you have to have insight into your students' world, their needs, problems, potential and aspirations. To that end you must understand the totality of the continuum of the teaching and learning environment – and you may need to be exposed to different styles of teaching and learning found in programme design and subsequent teaching and assessing techniques. For example, you should be open to teaching techniques that require rote learning, recall and repetition. Equally there is a place for teaching and learning where the students are self-directed and self-assessing. Finally, as teachers you will need to acknowledge and embrace the fact that educational programmes commonly incorporate a range of techniques and methods, all of which serve some of the learning outcomes.

Thus, assessment strategies say much about the nature, purpose and design of educational programmes. However, they are also tools by which teachers may judge their own performance and developing expertise, the success of the teaching and learning that have been planned and delivered and the means by which evaluation and modification may be implemented.

EXAMPLES OF ASSESSMENT TOOLS

In this final section I review a selection of assessment tools in more detail. You may view this selection as more (or less) applicable to your area of practice, but I emphasise that you should develop a general understanding of the scope, depth and breadth of assessment if you are to support your students fully in their learning experiences. Thus, you will need to apply the principles of these reviews to other assessment tools you may encounter. The tools to be reviewed are given in *italic* type in the general list of assessment tools below:

- *Clinical mentorship/supervision*
- *OSCE*
- *Practice portfolios*
- Reflection (in practice)
- *Reflection (on practice)*
- Diaries
- Competency framework
- Practical examination
- Practical exercise (observed/report)
- *Essays*
- Dissertation (a lengthy written essay, treatise, or thesis – research-based)
- Critique (critical evaluation of literature)
- Project reports
- *Written examinations* (seen/unseen, essays, multiple choice questions, short answers)
- Seminar/presentation
- Case history reports.

Each tool is reviewed using the standard headings highlighted earlier in the chapter:

- What is the assessment tool?
- What is the assessment tool testing?
- How valid is the assessment tool?
- How reliable is the assessment tool?
- What resource issues arise from this assessment tool?
- What other issues must be accounted for when using this assessment tool (regulations, professional requirements, safety, ethics, competence)?
- Preparation of the tool for use
- Preparation of examiners/assessors
- Preparation of students
- Marking and related issues.

BOX 5.5	*Clinical mentorship/supervision*

What is the clinical mentorship/supervision assessment tool?

Clinical mentorship is one of the most common forms of student assessment in practice – and therefore is a tool of assessment. For the purposes of this chapter the terms mentor, clinical supervisor, preceptor and clinical teacher are used interchangeably. However there are many important interpretations of these roles (Morag and Smith 2000, Bray and Nettleton 2007). It is important that you extend your reading and understanding of these varied educational roles in the practice environment.

The clinical mentor has unique access to the student's performance in practice, and therefore directly observes and assesses the student's practice. Such assessment is commonly based on competencies that students must achieve if they are to pass the placement. However, a particular advantage of the mentorship relationship is its flexibility in enabling either informal, formative and spontaneous student reviews, or more formal planned summative clinical assessments.

What is the clinical mentorship/supervision assessment tool testing?

Clinical mentorship is a tool that has two primary functions:

1. As a teaching tool – supporting, nurturing and developing the student's practice
2. As an examining tool – enabling formative and summative assessment of the student's practice.

The clinical mentorship tool is usually structured on a competency framework that is tailored to the specifics of the clinical area. It may be designed to test broad thematic outcomes (e.g. the ability to communicate effectively with patients and/or colleagues), or to test specific skills (e.g. wound management, medication management, injection technique).

How valid is the clinical mentorship/supervision assessment tool?

Clinical mentorship is, by its very nature, a highly valid assessment tool rooted in the practice experience of the student.

How reliable is the clinical mentorship/supervision assessment tool?

Clinical mentorship is reliant on the expert impression and assessment by the mentor of the student's practice activity. That intimate relationship between student and mentor may give rise to subjective influences. A well-designed competency framework, coupled with formal preparation of the mentor for the role, should enable an objective outcome. However, clinical mentorship is an issue that may raise questions of consistency and reliability.

What resource issues arise from the clinical mentorship/supervision assessment tool?

Clinical areas must be able to identify appropriately prepared and skilled practitioners to mentor students. In addition it is important that the student/mentor ratio is acceptable, and that students receive adequate attention and support.

What other issues must be accounted for when using the clinical mentorship/supervision tool (regulations, professional requirements, safety, ethics, competence)?

Students must be aware of issues of confidentiality when being assessed by mentors in practice and when accessing clinical documentation to inform their care. Anonymity in any written assessment documentation must be assured. Confidentiality is commonly an explicit requirement of employers, educators and professional regulators.

Students must practise within their acknowledged limitations and be aware of regulators' guidance on the scope of practice. Mentors must also be aware of national and local guidelines and protocols that guide and limit students' practice activity.

Preparation of the clinical mentorship/supervision tool for use

Clinical mentorship is an individual relationship between mentor and mentee and also commonly used as a tool to guide development. The tensions between those two components require that a mentorship-based assessment be carefully designed in advance and that the learning intention of the mentorship activity is transparently and explicitly clear from the outset.

Mentorship-based assessment is a continuous activity that may be marked by episodic formal assessment points. It is important that students are fully informed of their progression within a clinical area, and that key progression points are documented from the start to the finish of the placement.

Preparation of examiners for clinical mentorship/supervision

As highlighted above, mentors are the expert examiners in the practice environment. Thus they are both the student's teacher and the assessor of practice. This duality can cause difficulties when the mentor is presented with students who are underperforming. It is never easy for mentors to fail students. Consequently it is important that mentors are not only prepared for the objective nature of the teacher and examiner role, but that they also have a support mechanism to call on when difficult issues arise.

Preparation of students for clinical mentorship/supervision

Students need to be prepared for clinical mentorship, the nature and intention of the mentor's role, and the competency outcomes expected from any clinical placement.

Students will benefit from a structured programme of mentor meetings, planned (and paced) assessment activities, and guidance on associated learning opportunities that may arise in a clinical placement.

Students will also require detailed documentation of the expected competencies and standards as well as eventual verification in writing that practical competencies have been attained.

Marking and related issues

The potentially subjective mentor–mentee relationship is a challenge when mentors are required to mark or grade students' practice developments. This is particularly so when mentors have to 'sign off' student outcomes that will enable their progression or eventual practice as a professional. This carries a weight of responsibility for the mentor. This may be eased by the use of well-defined competency outcomes that should enable an objective assessment of clinical performance.

However, it is crucial that novice mentors have the opportunity to work with experienced mentors to develop and model their skills of mentorship and assessment, as well as receiving formal theoretical preparation for the role in accordance with the professional regulators' and employer's requirements.

BOX 5.6	*The practice portfolio*

What is the practice portfolio assessment tool?

Practice portfolios are increasingly popular assessment tools for nurses and other health professionals, and when properly undertaken they demonstrate students' active interaction with their clinical practice. Practice portfolios are a means by which students and teachers may identify broad or specific areas of developing skill, knowledge and competence during their practice experience.

What is the practice portfolio assessment tool testing?

Portfolios are varied in their design, but commonly require students to have both academic and clinical supervision and support. The student compiles a range of evidence from practice and collates this evidence with reference to theory and the research literature. The portfolio will ultimately document their practice, personal experiences, personal development and their competencies. Thus portfolios may include reflective components, practical examinations, competencies, essays, diaries, and other accounts and reports that underpin practice development. They allow the teacher and clinical supervisors to observe general and specific areas of the student's strengths and identify areas where students need to develop.

How valid is the practice portfolio assessment tool?

Portfolios are highly valid assessment tools. They can be designed to meet both general and specific assessment criteria, learning and competency outcomes. Despite that diversity they can be structured, are primarily student-led and based on individual and self-identified personal learning needs.

How reliable is the practice portfolio assessment tool?

It cannot be denied that portfolios are potentially difficult for teachers to assess due to the subjectivity of some elements, and that every portfolio is individual to the student. However, despite that, carefully constructed guidance and equitable support for students will enable a high degree of reliability.

What resource issues arise from the practice portfolio assessment tool?

Portfolios are high-maintenance assessment strategies for teachers as they require structured supervision from both academic and clinical staff.

What other issues must be accounted for when using the practice portfolio assessment tool (regulations, professional requirements, safety, ethics, competence)?

Students must be aware of issues of confidentiality when using practice portfolios, especially when including clinical documentation regarding patients or colleagues. Anonymity must be assured. Such confidentiality is commonly an explicit requirement of employers, educators and professional regulators.

Issues regarding plagiarism and authenticity may arise in portfolio work, and you and your students must be aware of the conventions and pitfalls and regulations.

Disability (dyslexia) – all educational institutions have clear protocols to ensure their students have fair and equitable opportunity during the assessment process.

Preparation of the practice portfolio tool for use

As stated above, portfolios are individualised assessment tools that can, nevertheless, be carefully structured. There is always a temptation to present portfolios to students as a blank sheet (put in what you want), but this is not educationally advisable as it gives rise to considerable anxieties in students who are unfamiliar with portfolio demands. Thus it is more usual to find a range of optional, suggested or required inputs. It is crucial that students have guidance and advice from clinical and academic teachers from the outset and as the portfolio develops. In the practice setting, learning contracts, competencies and self-needs analysis are useful mechanisms by which you can assist students in planning and structuring their portfolios.

Preparation of examiners for practice portfolios

Prospective clinical and academic examiners can be as perplexed by portfolios as students – and it is important that they have clear guidelines as to what is expected of them when assessing and grading. It is often expedient for new portfolio markers to work closely with more experienced markers until they become familiar with the criteria.

Preparation of students for compiling practice portfolios

Whilst completion of a portfolio is the student's responsibility, and forms a crucial aspect of their learning and overall assessment, they will benefit from exemplar formats or portfolio plans to guide their portfolio structure. For example, you may assist them in developing self-assessment and action plans, learning needs analysis, and provide them with clinical mentorship and supervision reports, clinical logs, reflective accounts or case histories, and perhaps evidence of objective structured clinical examinations or other practical examinations. You may also require that clinical supervisors verify in writing that practical competencies have been attained.

Marking and related issues

The diversity of portfolios demands that guidance is made available to markers on key themes and content that would be expected to be included. Equally, there is a demand that markers are either experienced in portfolio assessment, or are supported and moderated by an experienced marker.

| BOX 5.7 | *Reflection-on-practice* |

What is the reflection-on-practice assessment tool?

Today's clinical practitioners (from the novice to the expert) are expected to develop and have reflective abilities. In the broadest sense they are expected, through clinical supervision and mentorship, to reflect on episodes of practice, to examine such reflections and to learn from them. Reflection is concerned with a structured process of reviewing current practice experience, and evaluating previous practice experience following the acquisition of new knowledge and skills.

However, reflection theory is complex, and you will soon uncover a wealth of terminology and concepts associated with it. It can only briefly be explored here. For example, students may reflect *on* practice and/or *in* practice – and this may be an important concern for you in using an assessment tool.

What is the reflection-on-practice tool testing?

Reflection is a multifaceted assessment tool, not just a written exercise. In simple terms, reflection is a structured, critical and thorough self-assessment exercise. Students may use reflection on practice to describe, explore, analyse, conclude and learn from practice exposure. It is a tool that allows students to examine their actions, skills and feelings, and communicate those to supervisors and peers. Thus it is an interactive and effective means by which student and teacher may identify strengths and learning needs, and consequently enhance the student's professional development.

How valid is the reflection-on-practice assessment tool?

Reflection on practice is a highly valid assessment tool. However, it is also a highly personal (and potentially subjective) process, and you (the teacher) must understand that reflection is not a process that will necessarily lead to 'right' or 'wrong' answers from the student. In addition, there is a tendency for students to reflect on 'negative' rather than 'positive' clinical experiences, and the facilitators of such reflections must understand that reflection may not result in closure or conclusion of such experiences.

How reliable is the reflection-on-practice assessment tool?

Reflection on practice is an individual process. There are numerous well-documented models of reflection that are commonly promoted as guiding the reflective process (Schon 1996, Boud and Walker 1998, Clegg et al. 2002, Bourner et al. 2004, Moon 2004). This standardisation of process (use of reflective models) gives rise to reliability.

What resource issues arise from this assessment tool?

Reflection on practice is a high-maintenance assessment strategy for teachers, particularly when dealing with students unfamiliar with reflective techniques, as it requires introductory theory, formative development and a structured supervision demand from both academic and clinical staff. In addition, reflection-on-practice supervisors and facilitators must be adequately skilled and experienced in facilitating this assessment tool for their students.

Issues regarding plagiarism and authenticity have been identified in reflective work, and you and your students must be aware of the conventions, pitfalls and regulations.

Disability (dyslexia) – all educational institutions have clear protocols to ensure their students have fair and equitable opportunities during the assessment process.

What other issues must be accounted for when using this assessment tool (regulations, professional requirements, safety, ethics, competence)?
Students must be aware of issues of confidentiality when reflecting on practice portfolios and including clinical documentation of specific information regarding patients or colleagues. Anonymity must be assured. Such confidentiality is commonly an explicit requirement of employers, educators and professional regulators.

Preparation of the tool for use
As with the previous portfolio tool, it is tempting to give students a blank sheet for reflection. However, reflection is a learned skill, and in the practice setting where the reflective activity is based the teacher must nurture (as well as assess) the student's skills and abilities when using reflection. For the greater majority of the time it is advisable that the reflection-on-practice tool be based on an acknowledged reflective model, that students have opportunities to practise reflection formatively, and that they have examples of previous student work that they can use as a baseline standard.

Preparation of examiners
Prospective examiners of written reflective accounts should be familiar with reflective theory and process. It is important that examiners have clear guidelines as to what is expected of them when assessing reflective work and that new markers work closely with more experienced markers in the first instance until they become familiar with the criteria.

Preparation of students
It cannot be denied that students are often (initially) not fond of reflection on practice. There are many possible reasons for this: perhaps it is the requirement to explore personal feelings and self that many find intrusive or even artificial. However, it is also fair to say that once the technique and understanding of reflection have been acquired and refined, many find it a useful assessment process. The implication of this for the teacher in practice is that students have the opportunity to practise all reflective techniques (not just the written account), to have structured and informed supervision and instruction in its use, and be provided with careful guidelines on theme and structure.

Marking and related issues
The individualised nature of reflection on practice demands that guidance is available to markers on the themes and structure that the student has been advised to use. Equally, there is a demand that markers are ether experienced in reflective assessment, or are supported and moderated by an experienced marker.

BOX 5.8	*Objective structured clinical examination (OSCE)*

What is the OSCE assessment tool?
OSCEs are characterised by the objective assessment of a practitioner's clinical skills, based on agreed criteria, by an expert examiner in a predetermined scenario. These scenarios are commonly referred to as 'stations', and an OSCE examination may have one or many stations at which the student is assessed.

OSCEs can be undertaken in the clinical practice setting (with real patients) or may be 'staged' in an educational environment with actors who play patient roles.

It is essential that teachers who are assessing students in practice settings understand that they are engaged in OSCE assessment activity, even if this is integrated into, and a normal part of, daily clinical activity.

It is also essential that teachers in clinical practice are aware that their students may be preparing for OSCEs – and will need to facilitate practice opportunities so that students may practice (rehearse) their skills in the practice settings. The practice teacher is key to this, as are both mentor and clinical experts.

What is the OSCE assessment tool testing?

An OSCE comprises one or more 'stations' (scenarios) which may have patients (actors) and examiners present where students' skills and knowledge are examined. The number and style of stations may vary according to the focus, depth and breadth of practice to be examined. Thus OSCEs may vary considerably in presentation and structure.

Here are some examples of the range of knowledge and skills that OSCEs may test: interpersonal and communication skills, history-taking skills, physical examination skills, decision-making skills, problem-solving skills, interpretative skills, reporting and management skills, education and training skills, counselling skills, reactive (emergency) skills.

How valid is the OSCE assessment tool?

OSCEs are, by their nature, tools of assessment that test practice and so are highly valid. It is crucial that the teacher in practice establishes in advance what it is that an OSCE in the clinical setting is supposed to measure. There will be a requirement for evidence (written, observed, audio, video) from the OSCE examiners. This evidence will assist the teachers in making generalisations about the student's overall level and scope of practice.

How reliable is the OSCE assessment tool?

OSCEs may be criticised with regard to their reliability – their test and retest consistency. The practice teacher should reflect on the objectivity of OSCEs carried out by student mentors, and the potential for bias. It is certainly apparent that OSCEs in the practice setting must be assessed by clearly defined criteria and measures to ensure the results are accurate and consistent.

What resource issues arise from the OSCE assessment tool?

OSCEs require the presence of students, examiners and patients or actors. Thus, OSCEs are demanding. For educationalists there are many practical considerations to be accounted for when planning OSCEs. However, the OSCE in clinical practice (structured, guided and graded by the practice teacher) is no less structured or demanding in its preparation. Selection of the patient, scenario, time and place must all be undertaken and the student carefully prepared and informed.

What other issues must be accounted for when using this OSCE assessment tool (regulations, professional requirements, safety, ethics, competence)?

OSCEs warrant an entire chapter of their own in matters of preparation and resource. Preparing actors, ensuring de-roling following repeated examinations and scenarios, accounting for examiner fatigue and issues of safety (manual handling) – these are just some points. It is important to seek advice from other teaching staff when first planning an OSCE examination!

Disability (dyslexia) – all educational institutions have clear protocols to ensure their students have fair and equitable opportunity during the assessment process.

Preparation of the OSCE tool for use

OSCE stations may be developed from scratch, or may be drawn from existing banks of tested OSCE stations and scenarios. Developing and testing OSCE stations requires time and effort and will (should) involve the core teaching team and prospective examiners. A completed station will require information for students, details of the patient role and presentation, detailed examination criteria and pass/fail criteria. Stations should have been tested/piloted in advance.

Preparation of OSCE examiners

Prospective OSCE examiners must be individually and carefully prepared in advance of their scenario, and to ensure their skill and familiarity with the examination requirements. Remember that an OSCE examiner may have one, or many, students to assess in one day, and examiner (and patient/actor) fatigue is a real issue.

Preparation of students for OSCEs

Students find OSCE examinations intensely stressful. Thus it is also important that students are given an opportunity to prepare and practise for OSCE examinations. Student preparation should include: classroom role-play, mock formative OSCEs (with detailed feedback) and structured practice in the clinical environment.

Marking and related issues

When the OSCE is completed, all the examiners should have the opportunity to meet and discuss each student's performance. This provides detailed feedback from each examiner on the overall standard of each of the students examined. It also enables discussion and action on any difficulties observed or encountered.

Many programme teams will hold formal examination review boards made up of representatives of the course team, OSCE coordinator and all internal and external clinical examiners who participated in the OSCE. Each station is considered separately and the decision made (usually structured on predefined pass, fail, grading criteria) by the panel whether each student passes or fails that station. The profile for each student is then collated.

Note that you may be involved in helping with OSCE assessment at some stage of your teaching/assessing career.

BOX 5.9	*The essay*

Essay: what is the assessment tool?

The essay is a traditional, widely used but diverse and effective assessment tool that is useful in assessing knowledge and its application. Essays are written exercises that students complete in their own time (the student is given a set time for its completion and submission for marking). The topic, title(s) or theme is supplied by the teacher, and will be accompanied and underpinned by detailed guidance and taught content. Essays come in many forms – formative, summative – and may vary considerably in word length. Essays may be discursive first-person reflections, or highly structured third-person reports; they may be critiques, case studies, course work, dissertations or theses.

It is important that the teacher in the practice setting understands that students will commonly draw on their clinical experience when structuring and planning essays. They may draw on specific case histories, specialties, protocols and reflections that they encounter in clinical practice. The practice teacher will be instrumental in guiding the students in the process and should not view essays as purely academic assessments that are unrelated to practice.

What is the essay assessment tool testing?

The diversity of the traditional essay means that it may test many learning outcomes, and many areas of knowledge. The writing of essays is commonly viewed as one of the most efficient ways of assessing knowledge acquisition and demonstrating critical and analytical skills in the interpretation and application of knowledge to practice. Essays are also a mechanism for testing students' literacy as well as diverse organisational and presentational skills. More importantly, essays facilitate assessment of students' ability to internalise and conceptualise theory and articulate this to others.

How valid is the essay assessment tool?

Essays are considered valid tools when testing knowledge and when assessing intellectual and literacy ability. They encourage and enable students to focus on and develop skills of evaluation and analysis.

How reliable is the essay assessment tool?

When carefully developed, essays are reliable means of assessing a measured, rational, critical review of a subject. They enable students to present knowledge and evidence, and contrast this from varied perspectives. Essays are a tried and tested traditional tool that forms a foundation for many more complex assessment strategies.

What resource issues arise from the essay assessment tool?

Essays are popular with academic teachers due to their (perceived) relative ease of use, and their limited impact on resources. The teacher devises the essay theme/title and then presents this to the students, complete with a submission date. Of course, it is never quite as simple as that! For example, there are considerations on the level and extent of supervision offered to students during their essay preparation.

In addition, it is crucial that the students have a clear remit and guidelines for the essay work, as this will form the foundation for their effort. In reality, essays are time-consuming for teachers and it is important that issues of student support are thought through carefully in advance.

What other issues must be accounted for when using this assessment tool (regulations, professional requirements, safety, ethics, competence)?

Students must be aware of issues of confidentiality when using examples in essays of specific information regarding patients or colleagues (particularly case histories or reflective accounts). Anonymity *must* be assured. Such confidentiality is commonly an explicit requirement of employers, educators and professional regulators.

Issues regarding plagiarism and authenticity abound in essays, and you and your students must be aware of the conventions and pitfalls and regulations.

Disability (e.g. dyslexia) – all educational institutions have clear protocols to ensure their students have fair and equitable opportunity during the assessment process.

Preparation of the essay tool for use

It is important to have a clear view of what the essay achieves, and clear guidelines for the essay that have been seen and reviewed by other educationalists. In formal educational settings it would be a normal requirement that such work be seen by both internal and external examiners before being given to the students.

Preparation of examiners for essays

It is important that prospective examiners are knowledgeable in the area of the essay subject and that they have been prepared in advance, and supplied with the guidelines, for marking criteria.

Preparation of students for essays

Students vary considerably, from those who plan well in advance, to those who believe that burning the midnight oil two days before submission is a useful motivator! Thus, essay guidelines are important and necessary, and if possible, good examples of previous students' submissions are extremely useful to students in gauging the expected standard.

Marking and related issues

It is important that written examination marking is based on pre-set criteria, and that students receive detailed feedback from examiners.

BOX 5.10	*The written examination*

What is the written examination assessment tool?

The written examination has historically been, without doubt, the most common form of assessment in education – and is the assessment process most disliked by students!

Examinations are written/timed assessment exercises that come in many forms, both formative and summative. They may be structured as essays, as multiple choice questions, as short answer questions, or as a combination of all of these. The examination theme is set in advance and questions may, or may not, be seen by students in advance. Written examinations are without doubt good learning motivators and it is widely acknowledged that they have a galvanising effect on the most lethargic of students! They are also highly effective tools in assessing students' foundation knowledge and learning and are a cost-effective means of assessing large numbers of students quickly. However, I would be remiss if I did not say that they have many critics. Students are adept at playing the written examination system, revising selectively and exercising their abilities of rote learning and preparation of ideal answers.

It is important that the teacher in the practice setting understands that students will utilise the knowledge and experience gained from their clinical placement and experience when preparing for written examinations. The development of key competencies in practice will translate into the students' examination answers (knowledge of protocols, competencies, standards and current best practice and conventions). The practice teacher will be instrumental in guiding the students in the process of preparation for written examinations and should not view examinations as simply academic assessments that are unrelated to practice.

What is the written examination assessment tool testing?

Written examinations test foundation knowledge, the pool of information which the student has acquired and developed, and his or her ability to apply that to the question or problem posed.

How valid is the examination assessment tool?

Written examinations are an invaluable and valid means of testing knowledge (and memory!) The student either knows the facts, or does not! However, written exams are limited in their validity when testing cognitive application of knowledge and are not particularly useful in assessing affective (human) qualities. Most obviously, examinations tell you little of a student's practical skills.

How reliable is the written examination assessment tool?

The written examination, if carefully prepared, is an objective and reliable tool, where all students answer the same examination, in controlled circumstances, with predefined criteria. These criteria will enable the teacher to assign an objective grade to the student's work.

What resource issues arise from this written examination assessment tool?

Written examinations are efficient tools for examining large numbers of students quickly and relatively cheaply. There is, of course, a need for examination rooms and invigilators, but resource requirements are episodic.

What other issues must be accounted for when using this written examination assessment tool (regulations, professional requirements, safety, ethics, competence)?

It is important to acknowledge the known weaknesses of this form of assessment. For example, it is crucial that students are aware of what books or notes (if any) they are permitted to have with them during the examination – and the consequences of cheating!

Examination nerves are a common experience. For some individuals nerves can, if not correctly managed in advance, impair their ability to write effectively. This is a sensitive and difficult issue that teachers must identify, and that students must learn to manage.

Disability (dyslexia) – all educational institutions have clear protocols to ensure their students have fair and equitable opportunity during the examination process.

Preparation of the written examination tool for use

It is important that the examination paper has been seen and reviewed by other educationalists in advance to ensure a clear view of what the assessment will achieve. In formal educational settings it would be a requirement that exam papers be seen by both internal and external examiners before being used.

Preparation of examiners for written examinations

It is important that examiners are knowledgeable in the area of the written examination theme, and that they have been supplied with the guidelines for marking criteria.

Preparation of students for written examinations

Students should have the opportunity to see in advance sample exam papers and to practise answering questions in timed settings. Students must receive detailed written feedback on practice essays. Ideally they should also undertake a mock examination. This developmental work is important in the preparation of students for written examinations, which are seen as stressful events.

Marking and related issues

It is important that written examination marking is based on pre-set criteria, and that students receive detailed feedback from examiners.

CONCLUSION

A primary learning outcome for this chapter required you to describe the essential difference between teaching and learning. To that end you have had a fairly brief tour of the principles that underpin these concepts. I have provided you with a framework of learning and teaching activity domains and how assessment tools may be linked with, or arise within, these domains. You should now have a clear idea of the diverse assessment tools that you could draw on when designing assessment strategies and underpin this design process with guiding principles of assessment. I have also given you some detailed examples of specific assessment tools, using a standard framework to structure this.

I conclude this chapter by making two key observations for future consideration. Firstly, inevitably, assessment is something you learn in practice, and no amount of written wisdom is a substitute for the lived experience of assessing your students in reality in the classroom, or in the practice environment. That said, I would nevertheless recommend that you explore in depth the nature and theory that underpin your assessment tools and strategies. This chapter has only briefly touched on subjects and issues that warrant far greater attention, and this detail will be found in the educational literature suggested in the further reading.

Secondly, whilst I exhort you to gain practical experience of assessment methods, I cannot overemphasise that the assessment of your students is something that you cannot afford to get wrong. Teachers are often described as gate-keepers to professions, and it follows that if you assess your students inappropriately or incorrectly, then everything that follows may be flawed! The consequence of incorrect assessment strategies or mistakes in the process of assessing students is one of the most alarming and damaging mistakes that a teacher can make, particularly in healthcare education. Consequently, you must develop your assessment expertise with guidance from experienced educational mentors, curriculum designers, assessors and markers. I must also add that educational institutions (such as universities) have complex quality control mechanisms to ensure the proper design and delivery of assessment work. However, it never hurts to seek advice, and do your own homework – before you set your students homework.

REFERENCES

Boud D, Walker D (1998) Promoting reflection in professional courses: the challenge of context. Studies in Higher Education 23: 191–206

Bourner T, O'Hara S, Barlow J (2004) In-depth reflection using statements of relevance. In: O'Hara S (ed) Innovations in management learning. Brighton: University of Brighton Management Development Research Unit, pp. 29–40

Clegg S, Tan J, Saeidi S (2002) Reflecting or acting? Reflective Practice and Continuing Professional Development in Higher Education, Reflective Practice 3: 131–146

Department of Health (2004) The NHS knowledge and skills framework (NHS

KSF) and the development review process. London: HMSO

Moon J (2004) Handbook of reflective and experiential learning. London: Kogan Page

Royal College of Nursing (2007) Guide to advanced practice. Available online at: http://www.rcn.org.uk/__data/assets/pdf_file/0003/146478/003207.pdf. Accessed on 11 March 2008

Schon D A (1996) Educating the reflective practitioner: toward a new design for teaching and learning in the professions. San Francisco: Jossey-Bass

FURTHER READING

Arroll J (2002) A handbook for deterring plagiarism in higher education. Oxford: Oxford Centre for Staff and Learning Development

Boud D, Keogh R, Walker D (1985) Reflection: turning experience into learning. London: Kogan Page

Brockbank A, McGill I (1998) Facilitating reflective learning in higher education. Buckingham: SRHE and Open University Press

Clegg S (2000) Knowing through reflective practice in higher education. Educational Action Research 8: 451–469

Clarke A (1995) Professional development in practicum settings: reflective practice under scrutiny. Teaching and Teacher Education 11: 243–261

Cox J, Mulholland H (1993) An instrument for assessment of videotapes of general practitioners' performance. British Medical Journal 306: 1043–1046

Ecclestone K (1996) The reflective practitioner: mantra or model for emancipation? Studies in the Education of Adults 28: 146–161

Ertmer P, Newby T (1996) The expert learner, strategic, self-regulated and reflective. Instructional Science 24: 1–24

Girot E (1993) Assessment of competence in clinical practice – a review of the literature. Nurse Education Today 13: 1383–1390

Gray M, Smith N (2000) The qualities of an effective mentor from the student nurse's perspective. Findings from a longitudinal qualitative study. Journal of Advanced Nursing 32: 1542–1549

Harden R M (1988) What is an OSCE? Medical Teacher 10: 19–22

Harden R M, Gleeson F A (1979) Assessment of clinical competence using an objective structured clinical examination (OSCE). Medical Education 13: 41–54

Kettle B, Sellars N (1996) The development of student teachers practical theory of teaching. Teaching and Teacher Education 12: 1–24

Kolb D (1984) Experiential learning: on the science of learning and development. San Francisco: Jossey-Bass

Marton F, Saljo R (1984) Approaches to learning. In: Marton F, Hounsell D, Entwhistle N (eds) The experience of learning. Edinburgh: Scottish Academic Press, pp. 39–58

Rust C (2002) The impact of assessment on student learning. Active Learning in Higher Education 3: 145–158

Schön D (1983) The reflective practitioner. San Francisco: Jossey-Bass

Schön D (1987) Educating the reflective practitioner. San Francisco: Jossey-Bass

Selby C, Osman L, Davis M et al. (1995) How to do it: set up and run an objective structured clinical exam. British Medical Journal 310: 1187–1190

RECOMMENDED READING

Arvidsson B, Fridlund B (2005) Factors influencing nurse supervisor competence: a critical incident analysis study. Journal of Nursing Management 13: 231–237

This paper analyses the importance of structured theoretical and management preparation for clinical supervisors in the practice setting to ensure effective student development.

Calman L, Watson R, Norman I et al. (2002) Assessing practice of student nurses: methods, preparation of assessors and student views. Journal of Advanced Nursing 38: 516–523

This is an interesting paper that highlights the importance of careful implementation of new assessment strategies if they are to be effective, rigorous and reliable. This is with particular reference to clinical assessment of practice, and highlights the value of competency frameworks.

Hamilton K, Coates V, Kelly B et al. (2007) Performance assessment in health care providers: a critical review of evidence and current practice. Journal of Nursing Management 15: 773–791

This is an interesting paper that looks at clinical performance from the healthcare manager's perspective. It concludes that assessment of

clinical performance is reliant on multiple-method strategies.

Hannigan B (2001) A discussion of the strengths and weaknesses of 'reflection' in nursing practice and education. Journal of Clinical Nursing 10: 278–283

This paper provides a good foundation in the appreciation of the principles of 'reflective practice' with a critical discourse on the strengths and potential weaknesses of reflection.

Joyce P (2005) A framework for portfolio development in postgraduate nursing practice. Journal of Clinical Nursing 14: 456–463

An interesting paper that critically examines the use of portfolios in masters level professional education.

McMullan M, Endacott R, Gray M et al. (2003) Portfolios and assessment of competence: a review of the literature. Journal of Advanced Nursing 41: 283–294

A valuable discourse on the place of portfolios in assessing practice. The paper acknowledges the demand for a varied range of tools in assessment, and considers the potential of the portfolio to draw this diversity together.

Index